Practical Research:

A Guide for Therapists

Acquisitions editor: Heidi Allen
Development editor: Myriam Brearley
Production controller: Pauline Sones
Desk editor: Jane Campbell
Cover design: Alan Studholme

Practical Research:

A Guide for Therapists

Second edition

Sally French MCSP, Dip. T.P., BSc, MSc (Psych), MSc (Soc), PhD
Senior Lecturer, School of Management and Social Sciences, King Alfred's College of Higher Education, Winchester, UK

Frances Reynolds BSc, Dip. Psych Couns, PhD
Lecturer in Psychology and Rehabilitation Counselling, Department of Health Studies, Brunel University, Isleworth, UK

John Swain BSc, PGCE, MSc, PhD
Principal Lecturer (Research) and Reader in Disability Studies Faculty of Health, Social Work and Education, University of Northumbria, Newcastle-upon-Tyne, UK

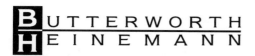

OXFORD AUCKLAND BOSTON JOHANNESBURG MELBOURNE NEW DELHI

Butterworth-Heinemann
Linacre House, Jordan Hill, Oxford OX2 8DP
225 Wildwood Avenue, Woburn, MA 01801-2041
A division of Reed Educational and Professional Publishing Ltd

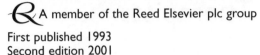 A member of the Reed Elsevier plc group

First published 1993
Second edition 2001

British Library Cataloguing in Publication Data
French, Sally
    Practical research: a guide for therapists. – 2nd ed.
    1. Therapeutics – Research
    I. Title II. Reynolds, Frances III. Swain, John
    615.5'072

British Library Cataloguing in Publication Data
French, Sally
    Practical research: a guide for therapists/Sally French, Frances Reynolds,
    John Swain. – 2nd ed.
    p. cm
    Includes bibliographical references and index.
    ISBN 0 7506 4620 9
    1. Medicine – Research – Methodology. 2. Physical therapy – Research –
    Methodology. I. Reynolds, Frances, Ph.D. II. Swain, John, Ph.D. III. Title.
    R850.F684
    615.8'2'072

ISBN 0 7506 4620 9

For information on all Butterworth-Heinemann publications visit our
website at www.bh.com

Typeset by Avocet Typeset, Brill, Aylesbury, Bucks
Printed and bound in Great Britain by MPG Books Ltd, Bodmin, Cornwall

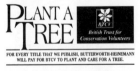

Contents

Preface

Over the past fifteen years therapists and therapy students have become more involved in research, either as part of their degree studies, or as a way of improving their practice. The need to justify professional practice and to demonstrate the efficiency of clinical interventions has always been important, but has become more urgent as health care practices and the use of resources have come under closer scrutiny. The theory and practice of the therapy professions encompass a wide range of diverse disciplines, from physics and physiology to sociology and philosophy. It follows from this that if research within the therapy professions is to be comprehensive and meaningful, it needs to embrace a wide range of methods and approaches.

The aim of this book is to provide a broad and practical account of the many research methods and approaches which are available to therapists, ranging from those which are highly structured and quantitative, to those which are qualitative and open-ended. It is emphasized throughout that no one method has a monopoly on 'the truth', but rather that each uncovers a particular type of knowledge. Ethical issues, the writing of research proposals and reports and the dissemination of research findings are also discussed. The book is designed to provide therapists and therapy students with the knowledge and skills to undertake research in areas of their choice.

This new edition has been extensively revised and extended in a number of ways. Several new topics have been added or expanded including clinical audit, participatory research, case study research and narrative research approaches. The book, which has been enlarged and completely updated, makes extensive use of examples from the physiotherapy and occupational therapy literature, and encourages active learning by the frequent use of 'Stop and Think' activities. These activities are included as a way of involving the reader and making the learning more active and interactive.

Every effort has been made to ensure that the book is accessible to students and practitioners with no previous research knowledge and experience. It should also be useful to more practised researchers who are keen to expand their expertise in new directions. The book is extensively referenced to assist those readers who require further information.

We would like to thank Heidi Allen and Caroline Makepeace for their guidance and encouragement throughout this project, Maureen Gillman for her contribution to Chapters 16 and 17 and Jo Laing for checking our final draft. Our thanks are also extended to all the therapy students we have taught over the years who have helped us to gain the expertise and confidence we needed to write this book.

Sally French, Frances Reynolds and John Swain

Maureen Gillman is Principal Lecturer in Social Work in the Faculty of Health, Social Work and Education, University of Northumbria, Newcastle-upon-Tyne, UK

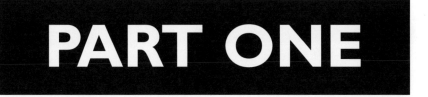

PART ONE

STARTING RESEARCH

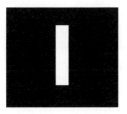

What is research?

What is research?

In this chapter we will be considering the meaning of the word 'research' and the usefulness of research to therapists. But before reading further, consider your own understanding of the term 'research', by reflecting on four or five images, ideas or feelings that you associate with the word.

Previous exercises with occupational therapy and physiotherapy students have shown us that students often associate the term 'research' with technical laboratories, complex statistics, and academic studies of limited clinical relevance. Clearly, these images and ideas suggest that research is difficult and far removed from therapists' everyday experiences. One purpose of this book is to challenge these assumptions, and to show that useful research can be carried out through small-scale studies, as long as they are well designed for the purpose in hand. In carrying out the exercise, therapy students have also reported a mixture of positive and negative feelings. Curiosity and enthusiasm are often balanced against anxiety and fears that the process may be 'boring' or 'too difficult'. Clearly, not all research studies will be of interest to everyone. Nevertheless, this book may help you to see that it can be a stimulating and manageable process.

So what is 'research'? The term can be traced to the Latin word *circare*, meaning 'to go round', gradually modified to *cercare* – 'to seek'. By the sixteenth century, the word in English represented 'a diligent search' (Onions, 1966; Skeat, 1978). These origins are important for they help to strip away the later ways in which the term has been mystified. Despite the many associations discussed above, 'research' refers rather straightforwardly to the process of systematic enquiry and finding out.

Systematic enquiry can be carried out through a number of different methods, and this book will help you to evaluate their various strengths and limitations. You will need to consider the research process carefully and defend your choice of approach. Different subject disciplines, or schools of thought within disciplines, have tended to advocate particular research methods, according to the type of knowledge that is valued. Researchers involved in the physical sciences (such as physiology and biochemistry), where causal relationships between specific factors are sought, have largely drawn upon experimental methods of research. In contrast, many who are involved in the human and social sciences advocate enquiry into people's thoughts, feelings or community norms, and regard observation or interview methods as appropriate. These differences have to some extent been reflected in the different research cultures to date of physiotherapy and occupational therapy. Traditionally, physiotherapists have aligned themselves more with the biomedical approach and have tended to adopt quantitative approaches, whereas occupational therapists have found qualitative methods more appropriate to their client-centred models of practice. Currently there are signs that both professions are increasingly recognizing the need to select whichever method is appropriate to their study. For example, the physiotherapists Mannerkorpi, Kroksmark & Ekdahl (1999) reported a qualitative study of patients' experiences of fibromyalgia. Occupational therapists have examined how purposeful occupations increase patients' perseverence with physical exercise through an experimental, quantitative approach (Hsieh, Nelson, Smith and Peterson, 1996). No one research method can be said to monopolize the truth.

Research methods are often deeply embedded within particular theories, which in turn are associated with different schools of philosophy or ways of looking at the world. If, for example, a team of therapists studying how people cope with spinal cord injury assume all difficulties stem from physical limitations (paralysis, poor bladder control and so on), their research is likely to focus on those physical limitations. The research methods that they select will, in turn, reflect their model of disability. For example, they may seek objective measures of independent mobility. If, on the other hand they analyse the difficulties in terms of the social and environmental barriers that exclude people with spinal cord injury from leisure and work occupations, then their research will focus on these wider social structures and barriers. They are more likely to adopt research methods which permit subjective enquiry into their patients' own experiences and beliefs.

These examples emphasize that there is more to research than 'fact gathering'. The purpose of research is to improve our understanding of the topic concerned, so there is always a theoretical dimension. The evidence collected during research always requires some interpretation, whether through a well-articulated scientific theory, a model grounded in participants' own beliefs or a sketchy, implicit explanation derived from everyday experience. Issues for research arise from discovering 'holes' in current understanding. This can be illustrated by considering some common stages in the research process:

Establish current understanding (e.g. through literature review, or reflections on professional practice), and determine what is unknown or uncertain ⇩

Frame the 'unknown' in terms of a research aim or question ⇩

Design a study that addresses the research question ⇩

Gather the relevant data* ⇩

Analyse and interpret the data – how does the new evidence

*('Data' – like 'facts' – are plural. A single measure is really a 'datum' but most authors avoid being this pedantic!)

5

extend or challenge current understanding: what further data need to be collected?

The first three stages form the basis of the research proposal. This vital phase of the research process will be considered in more detail in Chapter 4. Chapter 2 will present some strategies for developing research ideas and refining these into a researchable question. Most of the remaining chapters will help you to design appropriate studies, interpret your findings and critically evaluate the contribution that your research has made.

Why do research?

As a student or qualified physiotherapist or occupational therapist, you may question the need for research. After all, your work involves extensive contact with patients and clients, and a continuing commitment to keep up with developments in your field. These tasks take up considerable time and energy. Nevertheless, research skills and experience are increasingly important for professional development.

Stop and Think
Consider two reasons for therapists needing to acquire research skills.

For students, experience of learning about research methods, designing a research proposal, and carrying out a research study help you to acquire many skills and attributes, such as:

- The ability to think critically (about the relevant literature, about current practice).
- In-depth knowledge about a specialist area of personal interest.
- Creativity (in framing a new question, designing a study).
- Logic and objectivity (helpful for evaluating therapy practice as well as research).

● Presentation skills (which can be used in clinical practice as well as future research).

For qualified therapists, the above skills may be supplemented by the following considerations. Research experience will help you to:

● Establish and develop the evidence-base of your profession.
● Evaluate your clinical effectiveness.
● Justify the funding of therapeutic interventions (including changed priorities).
● Determine areas of previously unrecognized need.
● Develop theoretical understanding of therapeutic processes and outcomes.
● Carry out well-designed clinical audits.

In short, research contributes to major goals of the current health service, namely enhanced clinical effectiveness and cost efficiency. It can also inform knowledge about patients' complex experiences of illness and adaptation, enabling a biopsychosocial approach to health care.

There has been an increasing output of published research in the therapy journals by practitioner-researchers, and several examples are given throughout this book. Your learning will be considerably enhanced if you read some of the recommended articles.

Quantitative and qualitative approaches to research

Although many new researchers associate research with statistics, not all research involves quantitative, or numerical, data. Qualitative studies, for example based on interviews and observation, are now present in greater numbers in the therapy journals. The primary data from qualitative methods are usually verbal – the record of words from the interview or written observation schedule. The data may also involve images – for example, if observations have been recorded on videotape.

Stop and Think
Imagine that you are a member of a multi-disciplinary team that provides a 6-session out-patient back care programme for people with chronic low back pain. You wish to determine whether the programme is effective. Think of two relevant measures that you could feasibly take at the start and end of the programme. Can you think of a quantitative measure (involving a number) and a qualitative indicator (word- or image-based)?

Your numerical measures might include:

- Time taken by patients to walk a given distance.
- Patients' records of time spent in selected active leisure pursuits (e.g. gardening).
- Patients' rating of their back pain (e.g. on a 10-point scale, with 1 representing no pain and 10 representing maximum pain).
- Scores on a standardized test of independence in activities of daily living (e.g. Barthel Index).

Qualitative indicators might include:

- Patients' descriptions of their back pain before/after the programme (do the words that they use change in quality, or intensity?).
- Patients' diary records of their leisure pursuits during the pain management programme (are patients reporting an increasingly active lifestyle?).
- Written records of therapists' observations of patients' movements such as standing or lifting (are these tasks carried out more safely by the end of the programme?).
- Patients' accounts of their reasons for satisfaction or dissatisfaction with the programme.

These lists are not comprehensive and you may have thought of other measures. *Quantitative* research tends to view the world of phenomena in terms of *variables*. A variable is a dimension along which something specific varies. Straightforward examples are height, width, distance and time. The quantitative variables identified above encompass not only pain but also mobility, work and leisure participation, which are commonly restricted by pain. The complexity of the back pain experience has inevitably been simplified into a number of measurable components, each delivering a score. The *qualitative* indicators attempt to capture some of the complexity of the patients' experiences and therapists' observations, and may be more holistic. Rather than comparing patients on the same variables (nomothetic approach), qualitative researchers accept that participants will use personally relevant (therefore differing) words and examples (idiographic approach). To determine whether a quantitative, qualitative or combined approach is more appropriate for a study, some of the strengths and limitations of each broad approach need to be considered. Further information is added in later chapters.

Quantitative measures: some advantages and disadvantages

Firstly, consider the numerical measures listed above (together with any of your own ideas). From a researcher's viewpoint, what are the strengths of taking a quantitative approach to evaluating a treatment outcome?

Economical: Quantitative data generally take less time to record, collate and analyse than qualitative data.

Statistical analysis: Changes in scores (e.g. before and after the treatment programme) can be statistically analysed to determine whether they are small and likely to reflect chance factors only. Conversely, large changes may suggest that the programme is genuinely effective.

Comparing individuals and groups: it is easier to compare individuals and groups on quantitative scores than on their qualitative accounts and determine which individuals have responded most or least to treatment.

Participants' scores can be compared with norms: If a standardized test is used, then 'norms' (typical scores) may be available against which current data can be compared. Participants' performance may be shown to be within a 'normal' or 'impaired' range.

Disadvantages of quantitative measures include:

Over-simplification: the rating scale may not really 'capture' the information that is required. For example, pain may change in quality (e.g. from stabbing to throbbing) rather than in intensity (on a 0–10 scale).

Artificial: A quantitative measure may be simple to carry out in a research or clinical setting but it may have little application to the real world. For example, 'time taken to walk a fixed distance' along a level ward in a clinical setting, may not necessarily generalize to the outside world which has stairs, and uneven surfaces, nor to the patient who may be fatigued by carrying shopping in real life.

Restricts the focus of the research: Whilst quantitative measures have precision and address the research question, they pre-determine the nature of the data. Further relevant issues may be overlooked. For example, one major benefit of a back care programme may be to validate patients' health problems within the family and permit more open communication. This benefit may be overlooked by predetermining the focus upon a narrow set of variables.

Qualitative evidence used to be considered by some as unscientific and impressionistic. However, values have changed in recent years and some important strengths have generally been accepted. The qualitative approach views the world of phenomena as complex rather than separable into discrete dimensions or variables.

Stop and Think
Before reading on, consider some advantages for the researcher to collect at least some of the qualitative data outlined in the example above.

A qualitative study permits:

Insight into the participants' experiences: Central to the qualitative approach is the belief that people's personal experiences are relevant to their health choices and behaviour. Provided participants have no reason to lie, their accounts can provide insight into their coping strategies, satisfaction with treatment and so on.

The possibility of unexpected findings: Qualitative enquiry permits a more exploratory approach, and may uncover issues that the researcher has not expected at the start (e.g. unexpected benefits or problems with an intervention).

Understanding of individual patients' needs and responses: Detailed qualitative exploration of individual viewpoints and responses can help therapists tailor interventions more successfully to clients' needs, enhancing clinical effectiveness.

Continued development of the therapeutic relationship: Many therapists prefer to include at least a qualitative element in research involving patients in order to maintain a collaborative relationship. For some clients, such as those with learning difficulties, who have rarely had a 'voice' in past research, the qualitative approach may be particularly desirable.

However, the qualitative researcher needs to avoid certain pitfalls and limitations.

Stop and Think

Take a final look at the list of qualitative measures suggested for the hypothetical back care programme, and consider their disadvantages.

Time-consuming: Although time perhaps should not be a prime barrier to research, it commonly is (both for students and therapists). Transcribing and analysing interviews or videotaped observations inevitably requires a considerable investment of time.

Reliance on literacy and verbal fluency: Respondents' accounts vary not only with their personal experience but to the extent that they differ in their facility with language. For example, patients with a wide vocabulary may have more diverse words for pain.

Those who are used to written tasks in their working lives may be more forthcoming in diary records.

Patients may not know: Whilst enquiry into patients' own views provides an important perspective, patients are not necessarily aware of all relevant influences on their functioning, nor are they necessarily insightful about their degree of rehabilitation. For example, a patient may continue to describe the pain as intolerable, but yet be showing much less pain behaviour following treatment. Conversely, some patients, in order to present a positive image of themselves, may describe having a more active lifestyle than their relatives would recognize.

For further information on quantitative and qualitative approaches in research, see Chapter 12.

Validity and reliability

A key requirement when planning a research study is to consider critically the quality of the data that will be gathered. Quantitative researchers emphasize that valid and reliable measurement tools are vital. It is not always easy to determine whether your proposed measures meet these standards, but you should always explicitly consider these issues, from the project proposal onwards. The criteria for qualitative data are rather different, and so will be discussed later.

Reliability

Reliability relates to the consistency of a quantitative measuring instrument. An instrument or procedure is unreliable under the following conditions:

● If the researcher arrives at different measurements when measuring the same entity on different occasions.
● If different researchers fail to agree when measuring the same entity.
● If research participants give disparate answers on different occasions when working through the same test.

If the measurements and procedures used in research are unreliable, then the validity of the research is seriously threatened. Just as we are unlikely to have much faith in a clock which loses on some days and gains on others, we cannot rely on unreliable research instruments or procedures. In widely used standardized tests, the reliability has usually been well established. However, if the researcher devises a measure specifically for the research (such as a new questionnaire), the reliability will be unknown. It is quite onerous for all participants to complete a questionnaire twice so some researchers attempt to establish the reliability of their measures either by re-testing on a sub-sample or through piloting their tests on a different sample prior to the research study itself. The format and phrasing of questions can also affect reliability. For example, in long questionnaires, respondents may lose interest and answer more flippantly towards the end. Answers are more likely to be stable if the respondent gives a similar amount of thought and attention each time. Consider some reliability problems posed in the following exercise:

Stop and Think

A researcher-therapist wishes to establish whether patients with rheumatoid arthritis are less depressed following a treatment programme. Consider that the following measures are taken in the final treatment session and determine which are likely to be *reliably* measured by two therapist observers: (At the moment <u>do not</u> consider whether they are <u>useful</u> measures of depression)

1. Patient's score on the HADS (the Hospital Anxiety & Depression Scale, a standardized test).
2. Duration of patient's speech.
3. Number of jokes that the patient makes.

The pencil-and-paper HADS is scored according to clearly set out instructions. Hence two therapists with experience of this test should be able to give the patient identical scores. This measure will therefore be reliable. To time the duration of a patient's speech (and agree on the timing) might be possible with a tape recorder and stopwatch. The number of jokes would probably not be a reliable measure unless two observers could agree at the start what should count as a 'joke' and what should not.

Validity

Research requires reliable data, but reliability in itself is no guarantee of relevance or quality. Children with severe visual or hearing impairments may provide low scores on standard IQ (intelligence) tests in a highly reliable way, but inappropriate materials clearly do not provide a 'fair' test. Similarly, reliable measures of joint range and muscle strength may have little to do with the ability of disabled people to live independently. If you decided to measure depression by the length of patients' big toes, you would have a highly reliable measure. However, clearly this score would offer no clue to the person's mental state. In short, this measure would not be valid – *it would not measure what the researcher claimed to be measuring.* Validity, like reliability, is not easy to determine, but you need to screen all proposed measures carefully, and justify your choices. Look again at the above list, and decide which appear to be *valid* quantitative measures of depression.

Once again, the standardized HAD scale, through its extensive use in previous research, has established validity. To take one example, Glickman & Kamm (1996) used the HADS to show relationships between bowel management problems and depression among patients with spinal cord injuries. The other measures could *potentially* differentiate between the behaviour of depressed and non-depressed people but are also likely to be shaped by the social situation (e.g. a non-depressed group member may think it quite inappropriate to make joking remarks if aware that others within the therapy group are depressed). Opportunities for speaking would also be influenced by the others' behaviour in the group, affecting duration of speech. These influences would undermine validity of the proposed measures. Validity is difficult to ascertain. You may think it safer to select quantitative measures that have been used in previous research. If new measures are devised (such as questionnaires and rating scales) then the researcher needs to ask tough questions about which kinds of validity can be claimed. Various types of validity have been distinguished:

Face validity: the measure appears to have relevance and looks as if it is measuring what it professes to measure. This does not guarantee scientific merit!

Content validity refers to whether or not the test covers a representative sample of items. For example, a measure of patients' ability to perform activities of daily living that only scored independent mobility would lack content validity.

Discriminate validity: a measure with high discriminate validity is measuring something distinctive and different from other tests. Whilst depression is associated conceptually with low perceived control, if a questionnaire measure of perceived control provides profiles of patients that differ somewhat from conventional measures of depression, it would have discriminate validity.

Criterion/empirical validity is established if the measure correlates well with others claiming to measure the same entity. For example, Strand & Wie (1999) developed a test that simulates putting on a sock. They reported that the Sock Test scores correlated well with other assessments of activity limitation in dressing, demonstrating empirical validity.

Predictive validity is a variant of empirical validity; it refers to the correlation between a measurement and subsequent behaviour relevant to that measurement. In the study mentioned above, Strand & Wie discovered that Sock Test results correlated with patients' perceived difficulties in dressing one year later, establishing predictive validity.

Construct validity refers to the extent to which a test is measuring the underlying theoretical constructs. Take the concept of 'catastrophising'. This refers to a cognitive style characterized by dwelling on a problem (rumination), imagining worst case scenarios (magnification), and helplessness. Any newly devised measure of catastrophising needs to cover these three components to have construct validity.

Therapists should make every effort to improve the validity of the tests and instruments they use in research. Formally testing validity is, however, a daunting and time-consuming process which can become a major project in itself; it is rarely required of undergraduate researchers. There are many ways of improving the validity of tests and measurements, however, and these will be discussed throughout this book in relation to particular methods.

Internal and external validity

These terms refer to the appropriateness of the whole research design and the confidence that can be placed in the knowledge derived, rather than reflecting the quality of specific measures. According to Judd *et al* (1991: 28), internal validity concerns 'the extent to which conclusions can be drawn about the causal effects of one variable on another'. In other words, internal validity is high if we can be sure that our intervention, rather than extraneous factors, brought about the effect.

External validity is concerned with the extent to which research findings can be generalized beyond the sample of research participants tested. Interestingly, ensuring high internal validity can render conditions so contrived and artificial that they no longer relate to the real world, and threaten external validity. This is a criticism levelled against some laboratory-based research. For example, Heck (1988) attempted to investigate the effects of purposeful activity on pain tolerance during experimental tasks. College students' tolerance for electrically induced pain was compared on a 'purposeful' pencil-and-paper test involving filling in a grid of squares and a 'non-purposeful' control task of moving a pencil repeatedly around a single square. Whilst well controlled, and providing evidence that pain tolerance was slightly extended under the square filling activity, participants were arguably confronted by a high degree of meaninglessness in both conditions. Whether the results can really be generalized (as the author suggests) to patients with chronic pain in everyday occupations remains uncertain. The study does not clearly have external validity.

Some threats to validity

In addition to issues discussed above, there are further obstacles to achieving valid research data and interpretations:

Events not addressed by the study: Concurrent events in the lives of research participants may be responsible for the changes observed. Patients may, for example, become less depressed or anxious, not because of treatment, but because they are receiving more family support.

Personal change/development/maturation: Normal changes, taking place over a period of time, may be responsible for improvement or deterioration, rather than the effects of the research/treatment procedures. For example, an elderly person may show increasing confusion, despite intervention, from the progress of Alzheimer's disease. Patients may show improvements in functioning as their injuries heal or as they discover for themselves successful adaptations to their condition.

Test effects: Research participants may become familiar with particular tests, which helps them to perform at a higher standard. Fatigue, anxiety and boredom can result in poorer performance. Expectations and beliefs (including the placebo effect) may also influence participants' behaviour.

Selection of participants: Where participants select themselves (as volunteers for the study) or where sampling is biased through unsound methods of recruitment, both internal and external validity can be jeopardized. For example, if researchers examine the effects of aromatherapy or acupuncture on people who firmly believe in these therapies, then any apparent improvement could reflect a placebo response and may not be applicable to the wider population.

Loss of participants from the study: Longitudinal studies (that is those that continue over many months or years) are particularly subject to loss of research participants over time, through change of address, loss of motivation and in some cases, death. This can result in an unrepresentative sample, threatening the validity of the research. A diminishing sample can be a particular problem in studies of high-risk patients, such as premature babies. For example, Weindling *et al* (1996) followed up infants at high risk for cerebral palsy for 30 months to determine the effectiveness of early physiotherapy and found that

21% of the sample were lost through death and other reasons.

Social processes: Even quantitative researchers are now acknowledging that research involving people is never a totally objective, socially neutral process. For example, participants and researchers may be influenced by each others' mood, appearance, race and gender in ways that potentially bias results.

Determining the quality of qualitative research

Qualitative researchers accept that their respondents' accounts are influenced by context and other factors and cannot be 'reliable' in the sense of 'exactly repeatable'. Nevertheless the researcher needs to retain a healthy concern about the trustworthiness of findings. Reliability may be addressed in terms of the analysis process – for example, whether the researcher (or co-researchers) can agree on the themes within qualitative material on different occasions. Validity can be addressed in terms of whether the themes or meanings analysed are a fair reflection of participants' views. These goals can be achieved firstly through ethical, sensitive methods of interviewing, and then through checking the emerging analysis with the participants for their agreement (member checking). 'Credibility' can be sought by gaining sufficiently detailed material and by looking for contradictory themes that challenge the emerging hypotheses or theoretical perspective. The data analysis process should be carefully recorded so that others can check the decisions that have been made ('dependability'). Triangulation – the use of more than one method to address a research question – can also provide a means of checking the validity of findings. Mason (1996), Seale (1999) and Silverman (2000) offer detailed discussion of these issues.

Participatory research

This chapter has presented a conventional view of research as carried out by 'experts'. The researcher has been represented as making all of the decisions about what to study, and how. However, some types of health research now include service users in research planning. Some research has gone further in blurring roles between researcher and researched. Especially for marginalized groups, there is a great deal to be gained from being empowered to shape the research agenda and process directly, through participatory and emancipatory studies. This approach is examined in detail in Chapter 17.

Conclusion

In this chapter you have considered the meaning of research, its usefulness to therapists and some important concepts including qualitative and quantitative research, reliability and validity. All of these ideas will be revisited in subsequent chapters.

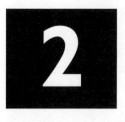

2

Developing research ideas

A good research idea will help to sustain your motivation throughout the entire research process. As you will almost inevitably face some routine work such as data entry or filling envelopes with questionnaires, a personal commitment to the topic is vital. Many students and therapists find the task of developing a workable research idea daunting and anxiety-provoking. Although there are no simple 'recipes', this chapter examines a number of strategies that can help you to find, develop and refine your research focus.

What is a 'research question'?

Humans appear to have had enquiring minds throughout evolution but not all of our questions are 'scientific'. Some questions concern philosophical or moral issues. Take as an example the question 'should all therapists have religious values?' This question could generate lively debate but it would need considerable re-wording to become a research question. 'How will treatments for people with Alzheimer's disease change over the next ten years?' This again is an understandable, perfectly grammatical question. As with the first example, it may generate lively discussion. However, it concerns the future which by definition is unknowable. The question cannot be answered definitely through currently available data and would therefore provide a poor start for a research project.

A research question must be explicit and focused enough to be answerable through an *empirical* study. Empirical data may be quantitative or qualitative, and consist of a set of observations or other practical evidence that can fill the gap in understanding that you have identified.

The researcher needs to be aware of resource and time constraints. Complex questions usually require a lengthy, well-funded programme of research. Small-scale studies need a tighter focus.

Selecting a field of enquiry

A productive first step when beginning a research project is to define the broad field of interest. For many undergraduate and postgraduate students, the field is very wide. The course may impose few restrictions upon choice of project topic. The position for employed therapists is often different, as research enquiries may be more tightly circumscribed by their clinical specialisms, and by the research agendas of managers and/or colleagues. This particular section will be more relevant to readers, such as students, who need to define a research topic from a wide set of possibilities. Later sections will be concerned with strategies for further refining the focus of enquiry.

As a student, it can be helpful to keep a log-book of questions, issues and references that interest you from the very start of the course. Such a record can provide an excellent source of research ideas. However, many students have not been encouraged to reflect upon their research interests until the time of preparing a project proposal! If there are few restrictions upon your choice of research topic, then your answers to the following questions may help you to narrow your selection:

- Which topics have intrigued you during your course (in academic and/or fieldwork elements)?
- Which areas have you studied in some depth, e.g. during a specialist option?
- Which areas of enquiry will make a worthwhile contribution to your profession?
- Which research issues are being examined currently in your

professional literature (or in relevant disciplines such as health psychology or medical sociology)?

Therapists who are considering starting a research project are likely to draw many questions from their work with patients. It is increasingly recognized that during the clinical reasoning process, therapists work through repeated cycles of observing patients and hypothesizing about their needs, progress and motivation. Their Why? How? Who? What? When? and Where? questions can provide the basis of a fertile research idea. It may also be possible to take a participatory approach by consulting with likely participants (e.g. a patient group) about their preferred research focus.

Certain restrictions are often placed around the questions that students are able to pursue in their projects. Hence, in addition to examining personal fields of interest, it is also important for the student researcher to ask the following questions, as answers to these will have a bearing on the topic that can be feasibly selected:

- Am I permitted to develop a proposal/carry out studies with patients?
- Am I permitted to research therapists' views and practices?
- Will my research data have to come from non-vulnerable samples, such as student groups?

In some courses, students' involvement in the research process is limited to designing an appropriate project proposal. Because there is no requirement to collect the data, the proposal can set out a plan to address therapeutic issues, such as treatment outcomes. However, in other courses, the assessment requires students to participate in the entire research process, including data collection and analysis. Research involving patients entails careful detailed consideration of ethics, and submission of the proposal to a local ethics committee (as will be discussed in Chapter 3) and students may be discouraged from attempting this approach to research. Examining clinical issues through research into therapists' views and experiences may be a productive alternative. Whilst such studies entail fewer ethical problems, they do take

up therapists' time. Therapists are therefore sometimes reluctant to participate, particularly in undergraduate projects. In
cases where students encounter barriers to direct patient or
therapist contact, and the course requires data collection, the
research question will have to be carefully framed to be answerable with a non-clinical sample. Such requirements are likely to
affect choice of research area. In this case, the student might usefully address the following question, in conjunction with those
above:

● Which therapy-relevant issues (of those identified through
  the processes above) can be examined in a non-therapy
  sample (e.g. students or general public?).

Answers may require some lateral thinking! For example, an
occupational therapy student may be interested in the effects of
creative activity on depressed patients. If the student's course
only permits data collection from a non-vulnerable sample
outside of clinical settings, the project may nevertheless be able
to address one aspect of the field of interest. For example, a
qualitative exploration of students' own reasons for engaging in
creative activity could be carried out, or students' knowledge of
the role of creative activity for a selected client group could be
surveyed. Such projects would still involve in-depth study of the
research literature on creative therapies.

Projects with student samples may also address educational
issues, so students may also determine their broad field of interest through answering this final question:

● Could the project examine students' *learning needs* in one of
  the therapeutic areas identified above?

For example, a therapy student may be interested in understanding more about the factors that give rise to falls in older
people. If the course does not support direct research with
patients (or therapists), then possibly the student could pursue
this interest 'laterally' from developing a survey of students'
learning needs in this area. There are many possible avenues of
enquiry, including a study of students' evaluations of the health

promotion/preventive aspects of the course, and recommenda-tions about how their college-based (or fieldwork) experiences could enhance their fall prevention work with older clients.

Selecting the broad topic from a wide field takes time and careful consideration. If you have located several equally inter-esting areas, then compare the practical feasibility of each. For example, you may be very interested in the role of genetic factors in rheumatoid arthritis, but research enquiry in this area almost certainly needs many more resources than are available to any small-scale study.

Another strategy for deciding between competing research interests is to carry out a brief literature search on each area. Topics for which relatively little research literature can be dis-covered (within a short space of time) are generally better avoided, particularly for a student project. In the absence of pub-lished previous research in the area, the literature review chapter of the project will be difficult to construct, and there will be little or no established guidance about appropriate methodologies.

Other factors that may influence decisions about broad research areas include the availability of:

- A suitable supervisor (what are the research specialisms of academic staff who supervise student projects?).
- Relevant library resources (for example, if your library does not stock specialist 'pain' journals, then a project on aspects of chronic pain will be more difficult).
- Student support (do you know another student who shares an interest in your chosen field, with whom you could discuss and clarify your ideas, and share journal articles, even though carrying out distinctive projects?).

Moving from the broad field to a more specific area of enquiry

Selecting a broad field of enquiry is the first step towards refin-ing the research aim, question or hypothesis. Most employed therapists and students conduct small-scale, time-limited studies, and these can only yield useful answers to questions that are well-focused. All questions reflect a puzzle, a gap in knowledge that we are driven to fill. Such puzzles may arise from many sources. Some are identified below:

- Personal observation and experience. As well as establishing broad areas of interest, personal experience, intuition and idiosyncratic observations can stimulate many worthwhile questions. For example, a student with experience of caring for an elderly relative with dementia may have noticed that certain environmental factors appear to influence the relative's levels of confusion. Such observations may lead to the development of a research hypothesis that could be tested through a systematic case study. Therapists have a rich repertoire of clinical experience to draw on when devising research questions, and they may have many personal hunches for why some patients respond well (or poorly) to therapeutic interventions. Perhaps one patient with multiple sclerosis is angry and difficult to motivate, whereas another with a similar level of physical dysfunction appears positive about her achievements and lifestyle. The therapist may hypothesize about the role of personality or social support systems. Out of such ideas may be developed a research question of considerable clinical relevance.
- Literature search. Theories and debates in the published literature may suggest new avenues of enquiry or hypotheses that can be tested. Particularly valuable are the final discussion sections of relevant research articles, in which authors usually outline the further research questions that arise from their current study. Although the research process is often described as a linear process, this is an oversimplification. In the preparation phase of the research process, there is a constant interplay between defining the relevant research literature and refining the research aim or question. As the literature review progresses, the researcher is likely to encounter numerous theoretical concepts and questions that were not anticipated at the outset. As the research potential of each one is evaluated, the literature search may move in new directions. Through the interplay between reflection and literature review, the student gradually defines the focus of the project.

The focus of a research study may also be defined through:

- Discussion with therapists or other students. Discussion can result in clarifying personal ideas as well as sharing questions and puzzling observations.
- Discussion with patients or users of services (including friends or relatives who use health care services). The views and needs of some groups (e.g. people with learning difficulties) are particularly under-researched, justifying sensitive enquiry. Users of health services often have a detailed knowledge of problems associated with illness or impairment, and may have ideas about how services could be improved, thereby raising many questions for research. However, the same ethical considerations apply as in research interviewing. Informal discussion should avoid intrusive questioning.
- Newspaper articles, television programmes and autobiographies. There are many feature articles on health-related matters (including autobiographical accounts of illness) in national newspapers and TV. Some authors have written books about their personal experiences of illness such as cancer or of caring. These 'testimonies' can provide a rich source of ideas for worthwhile research in the psychosocial domain.
- Brainstorming. Questions become more focused through being written down. Some students complain that their research ideas are vague and difficult to express. Writing down as many questions as possible on a topic provides a means for examining emerging ideas, and thereby the possibility of improving them. For brainstorming to be a productive activity, it is important not to be critical in the initial phase of collating ideas. Ideas, however half-baked or far-fetched they seem to be, can hint at the gaps in knowledge that the researcher is trying to define. The editing and evaluation of the ideas come later.

Final refining of a specific area of enquiry into a workable research project

Formulating your research idea requires time, thought and critical evaluation. You need to weigh up whether you are going to test a specific hypothesis which will need to be described exactly, or whether you intend to conduct a more exploratory piece of research. In qualitative research, it is acceptable to set out with a somewhat broader purpose than in experimental studies. For example, Trainor & Ezer explain the purpose of their qualitative research as follows: 'to begin to understand the experiences of men who were living with AIDS after having previously faced imminent death' (2000: 648).

Whether a hypothesis-testing or exploratory study is envisaged, it remains important to be quite clear about your aim. All too often, initially formulated questions are too broad to be answerable within a project's required timescale and available resources. The process of refining a research question is hardly ever documented by researchers, but Kamwendo, Askenbom and Wahligren (1999) provide an exception. Before presenting the findings of their study, they explicitly describe how their initial plan to investigate patient adherence to exercise programmes was modified to focus more narrowly on the personal meanings of exercise for patients with rheumatoid arthritis. In starting their project, they had realized that better understanding of these qualitative meanings would enable them to design a more appropriate study of treatment adherence.

Once the researcher has formulated a provisional research question, further critical evaluation should be carried out by asking:

- What am I really trying to find out?
- Can the question be broken into additional, more specific questions?
- Are the words used in the question clear and unambiguous?
- Can the focus (e.g. nature of the intervention, or sample) be restricted further?
- Can the question genuinely be answered by empirical data?

A question that includes wide, poorly defined terms is unlikely to be amenable to research. To explore this further, attempt the following exercise before reading on.

Stop and Think
Refining a research question
Some general practitioners have been prescribing physical exercise for selected patients instead of (or in addition to) medication. Imagine that you are a physiotherapist or occupational therapist working in primary care, and that you intend to evaluate the effectiveness of this form of treatment. You define your research question as:

Is 'exercise on prescription' beneficial to patients?

Evaluate this question, and redefine it in at least two ways to make the question more specific and researchable.

A good way of starting is by examining each term within the question. The question contains three major terms or phrases:

● Exercise on prescription.
● Beneficial.
● Patients.

Physical exercise encompasses many different activities, such as walking, swimming, aerobic dance, and lifting weights. Patients may be referred to a gym or fitness centre, or may carry out their exercise in their own home or local environment, such as a park. Whilst a large project might examine the effects on patients taking part in all forms of 'exercise on prescription', it may be more manageable for a smaller project to focus on the effects of engaging in one form of exercise, such as walking. In order to provide a fair evaluation of a group of patients, the duration and frequency of walking may need to be specified.

'Beneficial' is a term with many meanings. Again, a lengthy, well-funded project may be able to investigate a variety of subjective and objective effects. A smaller project will probably have to delineate more precisely which effects are being examined. For example, the research team may decide to prioritize pain symptoms. The effects of exercise on other problems such as fatigue, depression or overweight might not receive attention within a small-scale study. Alternatively, in a qualitative study, a deliberate strategy may be to explore whatever patients perceive as beneficial.

General practitioners may prescribe exercise to a wide variety of patients. Their assessed needs vary as do the objectives of the exercise treatment. The researchers may decide to focus exclusively on one group of patients, such as those with low back pain. Via this decision-making process, the research question may become more focused: *Do patients diagnosed with chronic low back pain report less pain following a programme of walking for one hour per day over 6 weeks?*

Alternatively, researchers attempting a somewhat more patient-centred enquiry may formulate a slightly broader *aim* (which of course can also be phrased as a question). For example: *To explore the perceived benefits and barriers to prescribed walking exercise among patients with low back pain.*

Stop and Think

Turn the questions below into more specific 'workable' research questions:

1. What are the benefits of horse-riding for people with learning difficulties?
2. Should therapy students be better prepared for working with terminally ill patients?

Each of these questions represents a reasonable starting-point for an empirical study. Nevertheless, small-scale projects (especially quantitative projects) may require a rather narrower focus. In the first question, the age range of the sample may need to be restricted, as adults may respond rather differently from children. Also the degree of learning difficulty (mild-moderate or severe) may be important. The nature of the benefit may be defined more exactly – such as balance, social skills or self-esteem. The frequency of the experience of horse-riding may also be specified. Thus a variety of narrower research questions could be formulated including: *Does weekly horse-riding increase the self-esteem of adolescents with mild learning difficulties?*

Alternatively, it may be quite appropriate to set out, in a qualitative study, to explore the benefits of horse-riding as perceived by adolescents with mild learning difficulties.

The second question concerning work with terminally ill patients, as written, is not clearly empirical. Questions which include 'ought' or 'should' usually express beliefs or seek value clarification. Regarding the meaning of 'better prepared', it is unclear from the question whose views are being considered – students, managers or patients, for example. Before coming to any decision about adequacy of preparation, possibly the study could attempt to assess students' level of skill in communication, say, for working with patients in difficult circumstances. Several empirical questions can be derived. For example, the research could survey students' or managers' subjective experiences or beliefs about the skills required. Alternatively, a more objective observational study may be possible (following ethical approval). As with the previous example, the level/year of the students may need to be defined. Two examples of empirical research projects relevant to the broad area of interest are: *What personal and interpersonal skills do third year therapy students regard as necessary for working with terminally ill patients?* And, *An observational assessment of the verbal and nonverbal communication skills of recently qualified therapists in an intensive care setting.*

Both studies would be likely to generate *implications* about the adequacy of current preparation offered in undergraduate courses.

Devising operational definitions

In addition to refining the research question through clarifying terms, as explored above, the researcher may additionally need to devise operational definitions of some concepts, particularly in experimental research. Operational definitions refer to the procedures and operations researchers count as measuring the concepts they wish to investigate. In order to measure pain, for example, the concept may be broken down into intensity, type and duration. One operational definition of pain may be self-rated pain intensity on a 10-point scale. Anxiety may be operationally defined by a standardized measurement (e.g. using the Hospital Anxiety and Depression Scale). The more abstract the concept, the more difficult it is to arrive at a satisfactory operational definition. Range of movement and muscle strength, for example, are far easier to operationalize than quality of life. With abstract concepts it is usually necessary to devise multi-faceted measures, as single indicators may have very limited validity. For example, 'patient adherence' (or 'compliance') could be operationally defined in terms of 'regular attendance for therapy'. However, this single measure excludes other equally important aspects of the behaviour. Patients who attend regularly do not necessarily carry out their therapists' instructions between sessions! They may have been forced to attend by a parent or spouse, yet none the less totally reject the advice given.

Operational definitions can have far-reaching consequences. If, for example, a therapist attempts to measure the success of a treatment programme, the outcome of the study will depend to a large extent on how 'success' is defined. Some people with spinal injury have commented that their therapists all too often operationalize successful treatment in terms of independent mobility, whereas the patient may judge success if enabled to re-establish former roles and interests (as noted in interviews carried out by Seymour, 1998). It is usually important in qualitative research to explore in depth the participants' own views about key terms and issues (e.g. 'stress' or 'disability'), rather than imposing definitions or making assumptions.

Starting with a hypothesis or research question

This chapter has focused upon developing workable research questions. Quantitative researchers often develop their project to test a hypothesis rather than answering a question. Hypotheses are clear statements that can be supported or disproved by the evidence collected. They usually propose that specific relationships between variables will be found, or predict differences between groups. Hypotheses can only really be justified when they can be derived from clear prior theory (and evidence), and they most commonly provide a precise starting point for experimental research (for reasons which will be examined in Chapter 11). For example, Munin *et al* carried out a randomized controlled trial to test the hypothesis 'that high-risk patients undergoing elective hip and knee arthroplasty would incur less total cost, and experience more rapid functional improvement, if in-patient rehabilitation began on postoperative day 3 rather than day 7' (1998: 848).

Strictly speaking, hypotheses can never be proven because the researcher cannot guard against future research showing the hypothesis to be wrong. It is safer for researchers to view their evidence as supporting or disconfirming their hypothesis.

Because qualitative researchers are willing to explore the complex personal views of their participants, and accept that individual perspectives may be very distinctive, it is unusual for them to formulate hypotheses. A research question is much more likely to generate an exploratory enquiry. For example, one of the research questions posed by Mahat was, 'What coping strategies are perceived to be most effective among individuals with rheumatoid arthritis?' (1997: 1146)

Conclusion

For convenience and clarity the process of developing research ideas has been considered in sequential steps, but in reality this is rarely how it happens. When, for example, the research problem becomes focused, it may be necessary to return to the literature; similarly, if operational definitions are formulated, the focus of the research may narrow or broaden. As was noted in Chapter 1, when using some qualitative methods it is both legitimate and desirable to allow some research questions to emerge as the research progresses. In general, though, your project is much more likely to be manageable and productive if you start out with a well-focused, clearly stated research aim, question or hypothesis, that can be supported by reference to previous research literature.

Ethical issues

What's the harm?

Sieber states that ethical issues relate to, 'the application of a system of moral principles to prevent harming or wronging others, to promote the good, to be respectful, and to be fair' (1993: 14). This definition centres, as we do in this chapter, on the traditional approach to ethics in Western societies, that is the use of general principles to justify and evaluate actions. The application of principles in practice, however, can raise deeply challenging dilemmas.

It would seem that concern about ethical issues in research has come to the fore with challenges to the notion that researchers are 'neutral', 'uninvolved', 'objective' and 'apolitical'. Researchers are necessarily involved by virtue of being human beings. Burr writes:

> No human being can step outside of her or his humanity and view the world from no position at all, which is what the idea of objectivity suggests, and this is just as true of scientists as of everyone else. The task of researchers therefore becomes to acknowledge and even work with their own intrinsic involvement in the research process and the part that this plays in the results that are produced. (1995: 160)

Researchers are also involved with other human beings. Research can mean intimate engagement with the public and private lives of individuals (Mason, 1996). Researchers have responsibilities to those immediately involved (including themselves), but also, as Sapsford and Abbott point out, 'those of whom (research participants) are taken as representative or typical, or even people who are not part of the research in any sense at all' (1996: 317). All research, from this viewpoint, is political, as argued by feminists and, as in the following quotation, by a disabled activist:

> As disabled people have increasingly analysed their segregation, inequality and poverty in terms of discrimination and oppression, research has been seen as part of the problem rather than part of the solution ... Disabled people have come to see research as a violation of their experiences, as irrelevant to their needs and as failing to improve their material circumstances and quality of life. (Oliver, 1992: 106)

Thus, research is not justifiable simply on the traditional grounds of furthering knowledge on the basis that knowledge is intrinsically good. A central challenge to researchers is the possibility that the essentially political act of research exploits vulnerable and powerless groups within society, furthering their disempowerment and contributing to their oppression.

Ethical concerns pervade research from conception, through planning and instigation, and throughout the research process to dissemination and publication. Though there are principles, there are no set rules for turning principles into practice. Ethical decision-making is essentially problematic, and a basis for reflection. As Sim states:

> Ethics in research is not a discrete entity but a 'conceptual framework' which underpins and permeates virtually every feature of the research process. (Sim, 1989: 237)

The aim of this chapter is to highlight the major ethical questions and dilemmas with which researchers are faced. Ethical issues pertaining to particular research methods and approaches will be discussed throughout this book.

Stop and Think

As a therapist beginning to get involved in research, it is most likely that you will regard research as a good thing: to inform and develop practice; to contribute to knowledge and understanding and so on. A starting point for thinking about the ethics of research is, however, the possible harm to participants that might result from their involvement in the research. List what you feel might be the main risks of harm to participants either in research generally or in a specific project you have been involved in.

Domholdt (2000) lists types of risks for participants in therapy research. There can be physical risks such as the development of delayed muscle soreness from the use of isokinetic equipment. Psychological risks include adverse emotional reactions to data collection in investigations of sensitive topics. Social risks can emanate, for instance, from a breach of confidentiality. The fourth category of risks is economic, such as lost working hours (including for therapists involved in the research). Prentice and Purtilo (1993) also list legal risks (e.g. criminal prosecution).

In clinical trials, major ethical questions are raised by the possible use of a control group. As Hicks (1999) points out, it is ethically questionable for a group of patients with cystic fibrosis to receive no treatment, even if this would in other respects be part of a good research design. She suggests that the research should compare two experimental groups, i.e. the new treatment is compared with the conventional treatment or another form of treatment.

Basic ethical principles

Ethical principles can be thought of as criteria by which decisions, procedures and conduct within research are formulated and evaluated. Therapy research, by its very nature, cannot be guided by a set of rigid rules which apply irrespective of context or circumstances, but by general principles that inform decision-making. The following are basic principles that apply to all research with human subjects (after Sim, 1997).

Beneficence

This is the positive requirement to promote the interests and well-being of others. The principle of beneficence states that 'we should act in ways that promote the welfare of other people' (Munson, 1996: 34). It is the ethical principle of 'doing good' which should be applied to the research participants, interest groups and also to society.

Non-maleficence

This is the negative requirement, not to harm others. Health care and therapy research can be 'invasive'. This is perhaps most obvious in physical procedures which may involve pain, but also includes procedures or questions which may be psychologically, socially or emotionally invasive. As Jenkins *et al* point out, 'both immediate and latent or delayed risks should be identified, as should any factors that might increase the potential risk for certain subjects (e.g. pregnant women)' (1998: 46). Non-maleficence means that therapists should neither intentionally harm their clients nor cause unintentional harm through carelessness. We would further add that non-maleficence should also be viewed politically, and as applying to groups of people who are not necessarily directly participating in the research. Research on a sample of single parents, for instance, can have implications for policy affecting all single parents.

Respect for autonomy

This is the ethical principle of respecting the self-determination of others. This can require the enhancement as well as preservation of participants' capacity to make decisions and act on them freely and independently. The violation of this principle 'for someone's own good' is known as paternalism.

Respect for persons

This ethical principle requires researchers to deal with others with due consideration for their dignity as individuals, and to value the inherent worth and uniqueness of each participant. You must beware of unjustly exploiting relationships which are unequal, for example those between therapists and patients, or managers and staff for whom they are responsible. Those who are most vulnerable, i.e. patients and students, may feel compelled to participate in a research project, even if they do not wish to, because they see the researcher as having power or authority over them.

Justice

All research is subjected to competing claims and vested interests, from those directly and indirectly involved. This includes the interests of researchers themselves. Ethical decision-making involves the recognition and negotiation of inherent dilemmas generated by differing needs, responsibilities, motivations and vested interests. The principle of justice obliges researchers to address competing interests at every stage, including the decision of whether or not to undertake research. This is the requirement to treat others fairly, irrespective of the researcher's interests. It includes the obligation to ensure that differential support, benefits and burdens are not provided for one group over another, including disabled people and Black and ethnic minority communities, or that if differential treatment of individuals does occur, it is morally justifiable.

Ethical controls

There are a number of controls over research and you as a researcher which you may need to take account of in relation to the ethics of your research. We shall consider five: professional bodies and codes of ethics; local ethics committees; peer review; education institutions; and legislation.

Professional bodies and ethics codes

Many professions working with people have codes of ethics or rules of conduct for professionals, including the conduct of research. It can be argued that an ethics code is an indicator of a mature profession, and therapists' associations have produced several codes including: UK Chartered Society of Physiotherapy (CSP, 1996); College of Occupational Therapists (COT, 1995); and College of Speech Therapists (CST, 1988). Sim (1997: 141–142) lists the useful functions of a code of ethics, including:

● The very existence of a code serves as a reminder that therapy research is a moral, not just a technical, enterprise.
● The code can indicate general ethical values which should characterize researchers' dealings with research participants.
● A code can provide a set of general prescriptions and prohibitions which may provide useful guidance for 'routine' decision-making in research.
● A code of ethics may stimulate debate and critical reflection by therapists on ethical decision-making in research.

Local ethics committees

You are legally obliged to obtain ethical approval from a local medical ethics committee if you intend to obtain a sample of users or potential users of the National Health Services through an NHS organization (e.g. hospital patients or those on a GP register). Each committee has a secretary who will provide you with an application form and guidelines. The secretary may also be able to supply the form on disc or by e-mail, making it much easier to write up your proposal. If you are interviewing NHS employees about their work, you do not normally need medical ethics committee approval, providing that the research does not involve identifying patients by name.

The form of a typical Joint Ethics Committee includes questions covering such things as:

● Project supervisor.
● The sample of research subjects.

- What significant discomfort (physical or psychological), inconvenience or danger will be caused?
- What particular ethical problems do *you* think there are in the proposed study?
- What measures will be adopted to protect patient confidentiality?

Applicants are also required to submit a research protocol (see Chapter 4).

Peer review

Research proposals submitted to a funding body and research papers submitted to journals can be sent to referees for review. Ethical considerations are likely to be a crucial dimension in peer reviews.

Educational institutions

If you are carrying out your project as a research student in higher education you should check your proposal with your supervisor whose name should appear on the form for the local ethics committee. Increasingly universities also have their own ethics committees from whom you may also need to obtain approval.

Legislation

The increasing use of information technology as a research tool spans specific disciplines and gives rise to a set of common ethical/legal problems. It is necessary to be aware of, and to work within, the law, taking into account such legislation as the Data Protection Act (1984/updated 1998) and the Computer Misuse Act (1990). Further, the unregulated use of the Internet highlights important ethical questions about the use of material that is deemed to be offensive and the limits of academic freedom.

As noted above, codes undoubtedly have positive value, nevertheless there are limitations, particularly as the research process is inherently fraught with ethical dilemmas that cannot be predicted at the outset and questions which arise in practice can be specific to the particular context.

Principles into practice

Whatever the usefulness of the ethical controls described above, the ultimate responsibility for ethical decision-making in research lies with you as the researcher. Furthermore, ethical decision-making is a process of professional reflection and judgement in therapy research not adherence to strict general rules. We turn next, then, to the process of addressing ethical dilemmas in the continuous process of decision-making in research.

To research or not to research

The first decision a researcher makes is to undertake, or not to undertake, research. In terms of ethics, this decision can be made on a 'risks/benefits analysis' (Prentice and Purtilo, 1993).

There are generally three possible 'beneficiaries'. The first, and broadest, is the general public and/or specific interest groups such as the research community, service providers and service users. The 'public right to know' is the dominant justification of conducting and publishing social research (Homan, 1991). Research which illuminates the detailed qualitative accounts of the feelings, experiences and views of individuals with learning difficulties experiencing problems in sexual relationships, for instance, is arguably justifiable in terms of public interest on the grounds that wider knowledge of the full personal implications of such problems may lead to the instigation of preventative and supportive measures to ameliorate such problems. As Sapsford and Abbott state, 'People may be harmed if their interests are not reflected in research, perhaps as surely as if they were physically or psychologically damaged' (1996: 322). There are dangers for participants, however, in that research that sets out to examine problems will find problems. The research might be used to restrict people with learning difficulties in forming sexual relationships (whether or not the researchers intended their findings to have such consequences). There is a danger, too, that the research may be poorly designed and may give rise to false data which, in turn, could be harmful to individuals, as well as hindering knowledge.

The second potential beneficiaries are the research participants themselves. There are many possible benefits for the participants, such as the opportunity to express strongly held beliefs. The third potential beneficiary of research is rarely mentioned in the context of justifying research, that is the researcher. Undertaking research can have many benefits for researchers themselves, including an enhanced *curriculum vitae*, enhanced professional status and publications. Much research by beginners is undertaken on initial training or in-services courses. Research can be part of the requirements for gaining a qualification. In this light, it could be argued that the whole process of justifying research is founded on establishing benefits for others as well as the personal interests of the researchers.

Respect

This principle seems unquestionable, but dilemmas and issues become apparent when research is seen as a process of intervening in the lives of others. Crucial questions here relate to the exercise of power in decision-making throughout the research. In this light, 'respect' is realized through the extent to which research subjects can exercise control over the processes of data collection and reporting. It is problematic to the extent that the power relations and structures of research are hierarchical, with the ultimate control remaining at the discretion of the researcher. Furthermore, there are a number of aspects of the social context which can further the controlling power of the researcher, such as a male researcher interviewing a female participant.

Informed consent

Informed consent has probably received more attention in the literature than any other principle of ethics in social and medical research. The principle is ostensibly straightforward – the research subjects' unquestionable right to make a voluntary decision of whether or not to participate in the research. It requires the decision to be 'informed' by an understanding of what the research entails, and it requires the capacity to 'consent'. The importance of participation through informed consent is, arguably, a safeguard to protect the rights of research participants, and also to protect researchers in fulfilling their responsibilities for the safety of research participants.

Obtaining informed consent usually involves providing potential research participants with an information sheet and obtaining a separate written record of informed consent. One way to view this is as a contract between the researcher and the participant. Informed consent is not required when using mail questionnaires (as potential participants can decline simply by not completing the questionnaire), but should normally be used when your research involves interviews and/or observation.

Your information sheet should be written in clear, non-technical language. All information should be provided in a form which is accessible and understandable to potential research participants. You should include the following:

- A clear title.
- A brief statement of the aims of the research and the methods to be used.
- A clear, accurate statement of what, precisely, research participation will involve.
- A guarantee about confidentiality/anonymity.
- Where appropriate, clear statements that non-participation will not affect receipt of social or health care services; and that research participants can withdraw at any time with no effect on services received. It may also be appropriate to provide participants with reassurance that they have the unquestionable right to withdraw from the research at any stage, and the right to withdraw consent to use any information they have provided within the research.
- It may be appropriate to specify any feedback that will be provided for participants during the research, such as research reports.
- A way of contacting the researchers.

In general, people should be deemed to be capable of making their own decisions providing that they are furnished with adequate information. However, there are some occasions when it may not be safe to rely on this assumption, for example with children under 18, people with learning difficulties, or people with dementia or serious mental health problems. In such cases, decisions may need to be made in individual cases as to whether an individual is capable of giving informed consent. In relation to research with families, Gates and Lackey ask, 'Are children's decisions to participate really their decisions?' (2000: 31) Informed consent is, however, clearly an important right. Explanations may need to be given in a different way, for instance verbally rather than in writing. Not to get informed consent from a participant can compromise the principle of respect for the person. When all other avenues have been pursued, you should normally obtain written informed consent from a person who is judged able to safeguard the participant's interests, wherever possible. This third party would normally be a close relative or an advocate.

Informed consent is not as straightforward as it may at first seem. With some research projects, validity may depend on the participants' ignorance of all, or at least some, aspects of procedures or intentions. To tell participants they are receiving placebos, for example, is likely to invalidate the research. Even the most respectable looking studies frequently contain some deception or other questionable practice. Educational research, for example, is frequently carried out without the knowledge or awareness of the students who are taking part, and the participation of students as research participants is sometimes a requirement of their courses. A neutral attitude on the part of the researcher to behaviour or ideas, which would normally cause anger or disapproval, can also be regarded as deceptive. In addition it is often impossible for researchers to give full information of their research; procedures, particularly if the research is qualitative, tend to emerge as a project progresses. Research methods and procedures do not, therefore, fall neatly into 'overt' or 'covert' categories, but are on a continuum where various aspects of the research vary from complete openness to complete secrecy.

One way round the problem of deception is to ask participants for their permission to be deceived. This is, however, likely to reduce the validity of the research, and may lead to a climate of suspicion and mistrust. Alternatively, an explanation of why the researcher found it necessary to deceive participants can be provided when their involvement in the research is over. Debriefing, with full explanations, can avoid negative effects and restore trust.

Privacy

Privacy, often viewed as a right, is a central concern in debates on research ethics. As a principle in social research, privacy is the right of research participants to control the information communicated to others, to the researcher initially, and in subsequent public documents of any kind. The central dilemma is, again, the rights of the individual to privacy as set against the public right to know.

Invasion of privacy violates a basic human right, but can also harm participants in more direct ways, for example by uncovering criminal behaviour. Haworth, in his guidelines for student research in occupational therapy, states: 'You will have to be fully aware of the complexities of the "research relationship" and ensure you know what is intended for public consumption. This may conflict with your goals as a researcher – to publish the "whole truth", for example' (1993: 9). The greater the sensitivity of the information the greater the need to protect the participant's privacy. Many researchers believe, however, that the invasion of privacy involved in most research projects is trivial when compared with the invasion of privacy experienced in our everyday lives. Ethical decision-making is complex when, as Punch states, 'there is no consensus or unanimity on what is public and private' (1994: 94).

Confidentiality and anonymity

Anonymity is offered in research when the researcher cannot identify a given response with a given respondent. In confidential research, the researcher is able to identify a given person's response but essentially undertakes not to do so publicly. While widely recognized as ethically sound in principle, confidentiality and anonymity, again, can be problematic in practice. Anonymity can often not be guaranteed. The more biographical details are made public, the greater is the possibility of recognition of the research participant. Anonymity and confidentiality also extend beyond the written word to include photographs, video and audio recordings, and raw data.

Issues of confidentiality can arise from disclosures made to the researcher and the principle of confidentiality can conflict with principles of safety and respect. Dilemmas arise for the researcher in situations in which the subject discloses information, for example that he or she is planning to commit suicide, which the researcher believes should be passed on, in the best interests of the subject or others. Recognizing this problem, Rubin and Rubin (1995) suggest that you should make clear any limits to your promise of confidentiality at the outset. We would also recommend that, at the outset of your research, you ask someone to be an adviser, to whom you can turn in the event of major ethical difficulties. This should be someone you trust with some knowledge of the area but who has no direct involvement in the research. It may be your supervisor, though he or she might be too involved. In any event your supervisor should be kept informed.

Ensuring that anonymity and confidentiality is protected throughout the research process, and beyond, can be far from easy. For instance, researchers may come under intense pressure, such as from parents, institutions or the courts, to release information. Changing the name and the gender of a person in a written report, for example, may not be enough and, in any event, opens up a new ethical issue, that of deception of the readership. Jenkins *et al* (1998: 49) suggest a number of steps for preserving participants' confidentiality:

- Any information recorded from participants should be kept in a secure location with restricted access, usually reserved for the investigators.
- Any information, photographs or recordings obtained in connection with the study that could identify the participant should be disclosed only with explicit permission from the participant.

- At the completion of the project all data should be placed in a secure location and destroyed at the end of the specified retention period. In some projects we have returned materials to the participants, such as audiotapes of interviews.

Safety

As we have seen, participation in research can be harmful in ways that may not be obvious at the outset. Research participants may suffer unpleasant emotions, such as stress, guilt or a lowering of self-esteem, due to the research procedures. For example, a researcher investigating honesty or altruism may provide research participants with opportunities to lie, cheat or 'pass by on the other side'. Participants must then go away with this new and unpleasant knowledge of themselves. Research participants may be harmed by adverse labelling, for example designating them 'non-compliant' or 'slow to improve' for the purposes of research. They may also be harmed by the indirect effects of research interventions. For example, research aimed at detecting high blood pressure may lead those so discovered to change their behaviour in harmful ways, such as becoming excessively sedentary. Some research may raise the consciousness of research participants to their own situation, for example to discrimination which may be limiting their lives. They may be very grateful for this, but, on the other hand, the newly found knowledge may create frustration, anger and dissatisfaction. Research participants may also be harmed when research projects end; elderly people in an institution may, for example, have enjoyed sharing their memories, week after week, with an oral historian. Once researchers withdraw, research participants may even regress. It is the researcher's responsibility to monitor continually the situation and build in safeguards to prevent harm whenever necessary throughout the process of research.

Exploitation

The final issue is the question of the researcher exploiting research subjects. The fundamental ethical question for researchers is whether their own agendas and motivations predominate over those of research paticipants. The relationship between the researcher and the research participants is usually an unequal one, with the researcher having more power and more knowledge of the research procedures and how the research will eventually be used. Researchers are therefore in a position to exploit research participants in ways which may be so subtle that they are barely noticeable. Researchers may, for example, unwittingly make it difficult for people to refuse to participate in the study, or embarrassing for them to withdraw. They may offer incentives which people find hard to refuse, or appeal to them to 'further science', 'benefit others' or 'help me through this project'. Research participants may also comply because they mistakenly view the researcher as an important person who has the power to bring about favourable changes to their situation. Researchers must be explicit in negating this misconception.

Research participants may give up a great deal of their time, yet the researcher gets all the reward in terms of prestige, qualifications and career advancement. Participants usually enjoy their role, but unless they are treated fairly and with respect the relationship can be said to be exploitative.

Conclusion

Ethical questions pervade the whole research process with dilemmas and decisions from the initial proposal to the final publication. Furthermore, ethical questions need to be understood and addressed within the particular context of the research. To conduct research is to become involved in people's lives. The experiences of research participants cannot be divorced from the responsibilities of researchers or from researcher/participant relationships. Ethical decision-making involves the recognition and negotiation of inherent dilemmas generated by differing rights, responsibilities, motivations and vested interests of all concerned. The processes of ethical decision-making should themselves be subject to critical analysis by researchers, and ethical issues need to be carefully considered in the methods sections of research reports and theses, and may be returned to in the discussion section (see Chapter 19).

Writing a research proposal

A research proposal (or protocol, as it is sometimes called) is a concise written plan of the research you intend to undertake. You will find it necessary to write a research proposal in a number of situations; you may, for example, wish to apply for funding, clear your research ideas with an ethics committee, convince your tutors that your research plan will work, or gain the help and support of colleagues and managers. If you are applying for funding you are likely to be in competition with others, which makes it vitally important that your ideas come across as interesting, important and viable.

The process of writing a project proposal results in three main outcomes:

● Clarity of thinking about the aims of the research.
● A feasible action plan.
● A means of communicating about the research with others.

Clarity of thinking about research aims: A succinct project proposal can only be achieved when you have clearly identified your research aim, question or hypothesis, and can defend this in relation to the literature. You will also need to think through and present the reasons for the chosen methods of data collection and analysis.

The research proposal as an action plan: A feasible, ethical plan will need to be presented, which includes a realistic timetable and resource requirements.

The research proposal as communication: The plan will need to be considered and approved by a number of outside authorities, such as ethics committees, grant bodies and academic supervisors. Therefore a concise and coherent presentation is required for an audience that may have little familiarity with the research area. In addition, the language used within the proposal may need to be persuasive, if the researcher is seeking funding. The people who read your research proposal will want to know exactly what your research is going to focus on, what purpose your research will serve, whether the methods you intend to use appear feasible, and whether you are a competent person to undertake the research. They may also require detailed plans and costings of your intended work and indications of the help and resources that are available to you, such as the loan of equipment, the assistance of a statistician, and access to suitable library facilities.

Structure of the proposal

Novice researchers often express uncertainty about the structure of the proposal. There seem to be few published examples (although you could examine the protocol published by Naylor, 1990, or Thomas, Fitter, Brazier *et al*, 1999). Perhaps because proposals contain original ideas, many experienced researchers keep them under wraps. However, students or therapists new to research may find that a more senior research mentor, or research lecturer, is willing to provide one of their own proposals as an example.

The required length and formats of research proposals vary substantially, so it is very important for would-be researchers to determine the requirements of the relevant authorities. This chapter will examine the usual areas that are addressed within the proposal, but academic courses, local ethics committees and research grant-awarding bodies each set out their own guidance. For example, some research grant bodies (especially charities) require researchers to include a lay summary of the research, stating the purpose of the research and planned method in terms understandable by the 'ordinary' (non-academic) person. This requirement is unusual in undergraduate and postgraduate research proposals. Some grant-awarding bodies specify the maximum number of references that can be cited, to encourage selection of only the most pertinent literature for the reviewers to consider. This restriction, again, is not usually applied to student projects, where a key objective of the literature review is to demonstrate the students' depth of understanding of the topic area. Although ethical issues need to be addressed in all proposals, those submitted to local ethics committees (for example, in connection with clinical studies) will require a higher level of detail.

The main sections of the research proposal

Title

This is often difficult to write and will probably have to be revised throughout the research preparation phase. It is important for the title to reveal the precise topic under study, without being too wordy. For example, although you should avoid vague titles such as 'Student stress', you would need to edit an excessively wordy title such as 'A volunteer sample survey of mature occupational therapy students with children to determine whether family stressors affect their academic performance throughout training: do third year students report more or less stress than first year students?' It can take time and numerous re-wordings to achieve a satisfactory title. In the case above, a focused but less wordy title might be: 'Managing course demands and family responsibilities during an occupational therapy course: a focus group study.' Note that a 'double-barrelled' title can be very useful as in this example. The second 'barrel' within the title can refer to the nature of the method (such as a survey) or can emphasize the exploratory nature of the study. Further guidance can be sought from the format of titles of journal articles in your chosen area.

Abstract

This is not required for all proposals, but an abstract forces the researcher to think precisely about the nature of the proposed study. Usually 150–250 words in length, the abstract summarizes the theoretical framework, research objective, basic methods and principal data analysis procedure (e.g. statistical comparison of groups). The relevance to clinical practice may also need to be made clear.

Introduction

This is not required by all proposals, but an introduction enables the author to set out the objectives of the proposed enquiry. This 'sets the scene', helping the reader to understand the direction and purpose of the literature review. The researcher may also give some personal or professional reasons for selecting the topic (such as observations in the clinical setting). For some research studies, it is also appropriate that the researcher describes his or her particular skills or qualifications for carrying out the study. For example, if the study proposes to explore children's experiences of physiotherapy, reviewers will be more reassured if they are told that the author is a paediatric physiotherapist with ten years experience. In brief, the introduction usually answers the questions 'What study?', 'Why this author?' and (sometimes) 'Why now?'

Literature review

Further details about the process of literature review are provided in Chapter 6. Most project proposals do not require a lengthy essay in this section, and the researcher should generally avoid (or severely prune) material which is only tangentially related to the question or hypothesis under study. The purpose of the review, from the reader's point of view, is to establish why the study is justified. You may identify limitations or flaws in previous work and generally establish the 'gap' in evidence which is to be filled by the proposed study. You may in addition need to examine the common research methodologies within the area under investigation, again to justify the approach proposed.

Stop and Think

Defining relevant literature

Imagine that you intend to carry out a qualitative study of how people with Parkinson's disease cope with their physical limitations, and you plan to compare the coping beliefs and strategies described by men and women within your sample. Which of the following areas of literature should you present in your project proposal? Omit any area that will only receive a passing mention (if any):

1. Research studies of the causes of Parkinson's disease
2. Current medical interventions for Parkinson's disease
3. Epidemiological studies of the prevalence of Parkinson's disease in different countries
4. Previous methods of assessing coping
5. Evidence about gender differences in coping styles or strategies (in Parkinson's disease or other chronic illnesses).

If the word limit is restricted, it is likely that areas 4 and 5 will be examined in depth, and areas 1–3 will be omitted or examined very succinctly, *and only in relation to the study.* For example, current medical interventions *may* be mentioned, but perhaps only to emphasize that in the absence of 'cure', people with Parkinson's disease have to find ways of living with their symptoms largely through their own efforts. Such argument and evidence would help to justify the project's aims. Whilst there is no one 'correct' approach, literature reviews tend to follow an 'inverted triangle' pattern:

Broad background to the study: e.g. clinical symptoms, major theories (briefly)

↓

Discussion of seminal studies related to the area under investigation

↓

Specific gaps identified in previous research

↓

The research question/aim/hypothesis

Research aim, question or hypothesis

This needs to be stated clearly, in terms that can be answered (or tested) by empirical data (as explained in Chapter 1). For exploratory studies, particularly those taking a qualitative approach, the broad research focus may be segmented into a number of more specific issues.

Method

This section provides a detailed action plan. It can be difficult to decide on the precise methods and analyses to be used at such an early stage, but to do so will help to focus and clarify your thoughts. Research is, however, a dynamic process, and sometimes researchers find their methods evolving during the study itself, for example through the piloting process. Flexibility of method is particularly valued in qualitative research (Marshall & Rossman, 1995). However, when researchers receive funding on the basis of their proposal, they are usually expected to implement in full the plan laid out. Hence it is important that the plan is clear and workable. The method is usually subdivided into a number of sub-sections, but some of these may be omitted from some proposals (for example, depending on whether a quantitative or qualitative approach is taken). The sections may be presented in an order different from that set out here. The researcher needs to consider their audience's need for a coherent 'story-line'.

Methodology: Not all proposals discuss methodology. Although this term is sometimes confused with 'method' it refers more philosophically to 'the theory of method'. The researcher may need to defend the choice of a particular research strategy as appropriate for answering the research question (Mason, 1996). There are differing views of what counts as a valid research method, linked to our beliefs about the nature of knowledge (see King, 1994 for one discussion). Methodological issues are most likely to be discussed when the chosen method is somewhat contentious. Whilst there is increasing acceptance of qualitative research into people's experiences of health, illness and health-care, researchers may still need to present a convincing argument in support of their selected methods. Nevertheless, it

53

is very important – especially when proposals are intended for an audience outside of a university setting – to present this material in terms that can be easily understood by people unfamiliar with the jargon, otherwise the researcher risks alienating the people who will accept or reject the proposal. Finally, where the planned research is to be carried out by a multidisciplinary team, different members of the team may approach the research using a variety of methodologies, in effect 'triangulating' on the answer. For example, an occupational therapist may be responsible for the qualitative aspects of the project whereas a physiotherapist may be responsible for the quantitative aspects. If a mixed-method approach is adopted (combining qualitative methods with standardized scales, for example) its advantages could be advocated in this section.

Design: This term is also confusing. It should not be taken narrowly to mean the development ('design') of questionnaires or interview schedules. Rather, the concept relates to the logical structure of the study. For example, are two different groups of participants being compared, or is the behaviour of one group of participants being compared in two conditions? Will the sample be drawn so as to support generalization of the findings? Is a single case study proposed? For reasons which will be examined in more detail in Chapter 11, 'design' is most often relevant to experimental studies. In such cases, the independent and dependent variables need to be stated, together with any variables that will be controlled in the study. For non-experimental studies, this section may describe the broad approach – e.g. a survey, observation, interview. If there are planned comparison groups (e.g. males and females, or more and less experienced therapists), this needs stating. In many qualitative studies, the researcher primarily intends to examine the experience of the individual, rather than make group comparisons. This can also be identified as a 'design' feature.

Participants: The people taking part in a study should preferably be referred to as participants rather than subjects (which connotes passivity). In this section, the process of recruiting the sample needs to be made clear, for example whether a random sample is sought, and the proposed sample size should be stated. In qualitative research, it is usual to state whether a random, convenience or purposive sample is intended. A purposive sample is not representative but rather is recruited to represent a range of different experiences. Within a small sample, having a diversity of expressed views may be more helpful for developing and testing theoretical propositions (see Mason, 1996 for further detail). Conversely, if the study attempts to reduce individual differences through inclusion/exclusion criteria, these should be made explicit in this section. For example, a study of postoperative recovery might have inclusion criteria such as 'female' and 'had a hip replacement in the last six months'. Exclusion criteria might be 'surgical complications' and 'over 75'. Thus the intended sample will comprise women under 76 who have had straightforward hip replacements in the last six months. (You are referred to Chapter 7 for more information on sampling.)

Measures/Materials/Tools: This section can have a variety of headings but essentially it describes the means of collecting data. If a standardized measure is adopted, such as the Barthel Index, the reason for selecting this measure over others may be given. The reference for any previously published scale needs to be included. A questionnaire, interview schedule or observation checklist newly designed for the study needs to be outlined. For more formal proposals (to grant-awarding bodies, for example) the proposed materials may need to be described in full. It may be sufficient in other cases to present sample questions rather than the complete schedule. Researchers using technical apparatus should give details (e.g. model or manufacturer). Reliability and validity issues need discussion. The important aim of this section is to provide sufficient detail for the audience to judge the appropriateness of the information to be collected.

Pilot study: A pilot study is vital for trouble-shooting the method, particularly for testing the suitability of the measurement tools or questions. The nature of the pilot study (who will be involved, how many, how will appropriateness of the method be judged?) needs description.

Procedure: This section sets out the practical data collection process in some detail. For example, that questionnaires may be circulated by post, with a stamped addressed envelope for return of the materials. In experimental studies, the order of experimental and control conditions, and instructions to participants will need to be defined. The location of interviews, and use of tape recording should be described. Procedures for gaining informed consent from participants may be stated here, or given under a separate heading.

Ethics: This section will occupy a lot of space in formal proposals to local ethics committees (such as those attached to hospitals or NHS trusts). All proposals need to specify the information provided to participants, and the procedure for obtaining informed consent. Generally an example information sheet and consent form should appear in an Appendix. Ethical issues, such as the possibility of harm to participants, need careful examination. Other safeguards, such as information giving respondents the right to withdraw from the study, and the safe storage of data in locked cabinets, require emphasis. More details about ethical issues are given in Chapter 3.

Resources: The skills, facilities and outside help that you have at your disposal should be explained. For example, a university may provide computing support, or the hospital may employ a statistician who will advise on the data analysis. It is essential, however, to get confirmation in writing from anyone offering assistance before mentioning his or her name on your research proposal.

Timetable: A realistic timetable needs to be presented, covering all of the tasks involved in the research process. Research nearly always takes longer than anticipated. If you are carrying out the research as well as holding down a full-time job, and/or running a family, your time will be limited and you will need to think carefully about how you can fit the research into your busy schedule. A 'cushion' of time needs to be included, if possible, to allow for unexpected difficulties and delays (such as failure of respondents to return questionnaires by the deadline requested).

Budget: This is a vital section in any proposal that seeks financial support, as costings for salaries, travel, postage and other expenses need to be accurate and fair, with each item justified. Students financing their own projects also benefit from carefully considering the costs involved, for example for stationery, printer cartridges, photocopying, postage, and travel to interviews. Therapists may need to consider the financial implications of time away from clinical practice, and research meetings.

> **Stop and Think**
> Cost of questionnaires
> Work out the approximate cost of sending out 30 mailed
> 4-page questionnaires, with stamped return envelopes.
> This involves 120 photocopies, 60 envelopes and 60 stamps
> so the overall cost may surprise you!

Data analysis: The likely approach to data analysis requires clear description. For qualitative data, the key stages of analysis should be identified. If a model is being followed such as grounded theory (Strauss and Corbin, 1990) then this needs to be stated and referenced. Further details can be mentioned such as the use of second coders (or participants themselves) to check on the trustworthiness of the themes extracted. For quantitative data, this section will present summaries of the descriptive and inferential statistics that are planned, with reasons for the choice of tests. This section requires considerable planning, but researchers who envisage their data analysis procedures in detail are much less likely to experience the horrifying discovery half way through the research that their data are unable to address their question or hypothesis!

References: As with all written work, you need to check that all references have been given in the required format.

Appendix: This may be used for sample questionnaires, information sheets and consent forms.

Curriculum vitae: Student proposals rarely require the support of a curriculum vitae (CV), but proposals to hospital authorities and funding bodies almost always do. The CV should usually be brief and well focused. The people who look at your research proposal will need to be assured that you are capable of carrying out the research. It is therefore wise to state your qualifications, together with all clinical and research experience that is relevant to the project.

Applying for research funding

It is advisable for therapists, in the first instance, to approach their professional organizations for advice regarding funding for their research. A variety of organizations publish calls for research proposals on specific topics from time to time in the professional journals, as well as in national newspapers such as the *Guardian*, and *The Times Higher Education Supplement*. Therapists may find that their research interest can be channelled towards the area specified by funding bodies. Sources of funds include government (for example the National Health Service), research councils (for example the Medical Research Council), charitable trusts and foundations (for example the Joseph Rowntree Foundation). Research fellowships and studentships are also sometimes available, although these often require a full-time commitment to the research. Therapists may also consider whether their research area would be of interest to industry, and seek business sponsorship. The further suggestions presented by the English National Board for Nursing (1998) have relevance to physiotherapists and occupational therapists.

When funds are so hard to come by it may seem inappropriate to talk about choosing a funding body. Therapists cannot, however, escape the ethical issues which arise when considering the acceptance of funds from different organizations. They may, for example, dislike the idea of accepting money from certain drug companies, from charities whose views and practices do not accord with their own, or from companies with political connections of which they disapprove. It is important that therapists' values are in accord with their sponsors because there is an unequal power relationship and researchers are often compelled to comply with the ideas of their sponsors regarding the content, methods and analysis of the research. Although values are slowly changing, it still seems easier to receive funding for quantitative projects that yield statistical outcomes than for qualitative studies.

Conclusion

Research proposals are not easy to write, as the process forces researchers to think in detail about their research at a very early stage. Nevertheless the development and acceptance of a proposal is the first step to answering the question that the researcher has in mind. When produced as a multi-disciplinary team effort, the process can cement the group as a working unit and can help members appreciate the resources that each person brings to the research effort. Finalising a proposal can be a creative and exciting problem-solving experience.

Working with others

You're not alone

As evident in other chapters, research is best conceived as a collaborative activity, from start to finish, from conception and planning to publication. Prospective research students who think of research as something they undertake independently, working alone, can feel so daunted that they never begin. As discussed in Chapter 17, a participative approach can be taken which involves researching with participants rather than on 'research subjects'. It is also possible to approach research as a group or team rather than an individual exercise. This is most often referred to as a collaborative approach to research. Collaboration has many potential benefits for beginners to research. Support can keep up morale during a lengthy research project and provide help in the complex choices that sometimes have to be made.

Stop and Think
Perhaps the first question is with whom to work. Who might you work with on a research project? Though it may be difficult to think in the abstract, rather than with a specific project in mind, make a list of people you might consider working with on a research project.

Your list will, of course, depend on the specific context in which you are working, however you might have mentioned people from three groups.

1. If you are a research student you might have listed people at the higher education institution including fellow students, lecturers and, most particularly, research supervisors.
2. Research is often undertaken by a multiprofessional team of researchers, including those within education and social work, and medical and paramedical professionals.
3. There is a broader group of possible experts, such as statisticians, who can be consulted by a researcher.

Working with supervisors

Anyone new to research would be well advised to work with a supervisor, or mentor, who has research experience. Seale and Barnard go so far as to suggest that you should 'never start a research project without some form of support system' (1998: 159). You should consider yourself as learning as much about the whole research process as about whatever you are researching. In many degree programmes, at undergraduate and masters level, a major purpose of the research component is to enable students to learn about the research process, as well as to study a research topic in depth. Effective supervision can be crucial in this. Usually the supervision is provided by an academic (or academics) from an educational institution, particularly when the research is part of a professional qualification course or for the presentation of a dissertation for a higher degree. Phillips and Pugh advise students to 'be aware that you must accept the responsibility for managing the relationship between you and your supervisor. It is too important to be left to chance' (1994: 111). Here we explore this relationship and your part in its management.

Perhaps the first thing to consider is what supervision has to offer. Thompson lists the following possible benefits of supervision. Does this reflect your experiences?

- Opportunity to share concerns.

- A forum for reviewing actions and checking plans.
- A more objective perspective on your work.
- Constructive feedback, both positive and negative.
- A source of confidence and reassurance.
- Opportunities for personal and professional development. (1996: 49).

The processes of supervision are, of course, of primary importance. A framework of general forms of helping suggests four possible models of the research student–supervisor relationship: telling, advising, diagnosing and prescribing, and collegial (Swain, 1995). The first, *telling* model, involves the supervisor as expert passing on his or her skills or expertise to the apprentice researcher. The second, *advising*, again involves the passing on of information, drawn from his or her expertise, but more in terms of suggesting possible options or alternatives from which the student might choose. *Diagnosing and prescribing* involves the supervisor in diagnosing the needs of the student in terms of progress within the research and then prescribing the best way forward in becoming a researcher. The fourth is the *collegial* model. Jenkins *et al* explain:

> the student and supervisor (are) engaged in a joint endeavour. As an adult learner, the research student is empowered with a degree of autonomy and is accepted into the research community. In the collegial model there is a degree of equity and mutual responsibility, and therefore control is shared between the supervisor and the student. (1998: 65)

Whilst each of these models of helping can play a part in research supervision at some stage, the collegial offers the best basis for student–supervisor relationships. Many factors will influence the progress of supervision, not least the expectations of the participants and whether the student and supervisor are both drawing on the same model of supervision.

What might your supervisor do? The responsibilities of your supervisor will usually include the following:

- Establishing, at the beginning of the research, a framework

for supervision, including arrangements for regular supervisory meetings.
- Defining the role of each supervisor, if there is joint supervision.
- Meeting you regularly and frequently.
- Giving assistance on defining the topic of research.
- Making sure that the project:
  Falls within the supervisor's area of expertise
  Can be completed with the resources available
  Can be completed within the prescribed period of study
  Is suitable for the degree being taken
  Where applicable, can be completed within the period of the studentship.
- Making sure that you know about research training provided by the university.

Stop and Think

What might supervisors reasonably expect of their students? Make a list of what a supervisor might expect of you (either from direct experience of working with a supervisor, or from general expectations).

The following list is from an Open University leaflet called, *Code of Practice for Supervisors and Research*. We have added to this using a list of what supervisors expect of their doctoral students suggested by Phillips and Pugh (1994) on the basis of a study they conducted.

- Produce a substantial amount of written work (not just a first draft).
- Tell them about other people with whom they discuss their work.
- Discuss with their supervisor the form of help which they need.
- Take the initiative in raising problems or difficulties.
- Recognize that their supervisor may have other demands on his or her time.

- Be independent.
- Have regular supervision meetings.
- Be honest when reporting on progress.
- Follow the supervisor's advice.
- Produce progress reports to which feedback can be provided by the supervisor.
- Be excited about the work, able to surprise their supervisor and be fun to be with!

There are a number of options for students wishing to make the most effective use of supervision (Thompson, 1996):

Consult the institution guidelines: If you are undertaking a course or research degree in higher education, you should be familiar with the institution's guidance and procedures for candidates and supervisors, which can specify such things as membership of supervision teams and complaints procedures.

Avoid 'macho' attitudes: This can be a barrier and sometimes derives from the belief that research is an independent activity, thus to require supervision, or help of any kind, can be seen as a sign of weakness. Researchers can be particularly sensitive to comments on their written work – as we know from both sides of the relationship. As we shall discuss in Chapter 19, writing is best seen as being developed over time and several drafts. Difficulties can occur when the student, or indeed supervisor, expects consummation with the first draft. The effectiveness of supervision depends, in part, on the student being open and receptive to support and help.

Ensure you receive supervision: If, for whatever reason, student–supervisor contact is difficult to maintain, the student can be proactive in receiving supervision. You might, for instance, send questions in writing; make contact in different ways, e.g. via e-mail; and discuss your supervision with your supervisor.

Prepare for and keep a record of meetings: For instance, a list of questions can be a useful starting point for a meeting with the supervisor. Some students also find it useful to make notes during a meeting (or even tape-record the session) or to write up the session afterwards. It can also be useful to provide your supervisor with a copy of the notes, or write-up, so that he or she knows how you perceived the session, and what aspects were helpful.

Identify your own needs: It can be helpful to both you and your supervisor if you identify what you need from supervision. This, we have found, can change over the period of the research.

The frequency, duration and content of supervision meetings the research student needs, and also that the supervisor is able to provide, should be addressed. This can include the possibility of access to the supervisor outside scheduled meeting times. Furthermore, there can be a supervisory and advisory team and attention needs to be given to the specific roles of each supervisor and advisor. For instance, we have worked in teams in which one of the supervisors concentrated more on the research methodology and had little knowledge of the substantive focus of the research. Attention needs to be given, too, to the organization and co-ordination of support, including who attends meetings, the focus and content of meetings and the communication between student and supervisors, and between supervisors. There are a number of strategies you might adopt if you have more than one supervisor (Phillips and Pugh, 1994: 111). A preliminary joint meeting is important at which you and the supervising team can discuss how the project will develop. Such joint meetings should be arranged at regular intervals. It will be useful too if the supervisors have (at the very least) telephone contact with each other once a semester. You should always send each supervisor a copy of what you are currently writing but make it clear whether it is for 'information only' or 'for comments'. Essentially you need to keep each supervisor informed of what you are doing and how the supervisory team is responding to your work.

A major set of issues for the student and the team as a whole can be the handling of the student's personal circumstances. One of us (J.S.) supervised a student who faced a particularly difficult set of circumstances in her personal and professional life. This student had totally to change her research project, with support from her supervisor, and the final project took her five years rather than the projected one year. Though this was an extreme case, we would suggest both students and supervisors need to be aware of the specific purposes of supervision, and it may be necessary to see research supervision within a broader framework of student services.

Whatever the strengths of the supervision team, it can be advisable to seek the advice of other experts in research design at different stages during the project. These experts may include a statistician, epidemiologist, a computer programmer, librarians and lay people. You might, for instance, need advice at the stage of developing the proposal, such as suggestions for preliminary reading, selection of the statistical model to be applied to test any hypotheses and calculations of required sample size.

Working in teams

Many therapists become involved in research by working as part of a team. This, of course, reflects the multidisciplinary contexts in which many therapists work. Such teams can take many forms, including for instance a group of undergraduate or postgraduate students under the supervision of a member of academic staff. There are many potential benefits to working in a research team, including sharing the workload, negotiating shared understanding from different perspectives and combining resources and networks. There can also, of course, be difficulties. Punch emphazises the possibilities for conflict which may be particularly pertinent for those who begin their research experience by working with a team:

> In team research, leadership, supervision, discipline, morale, status, salaries, careers prospects, and the intellectual division of labor can promote unexpected tensions in the field ... Workloads, ownership of data, rights of publication, and career and status issues are all affected by the constraints of team research. (1998: 164)

Miller also states:

> The process of bringing together people with different languages, different assumptions about ways of knowing, different conceptual

frameworks, different values and different bases for their career success in order to engage an identified problem seems intimidating. (1994: 266)

Teams can take many different forms. Gilkeson (1997), for instance, distinguishes between multidisciplinary and interdisciplinary teamwork. The former is characterized by a juxtaposition of professions from different disciplines, working side by side, each separately bringing their own expertise to the problem. Interdisciplinary teamwork, however, is characterized by 'intense co-operation centered on a common problem-solving purpose' (p 99). Laidler (1994) considers two features as necessary to achieve interdisciplinary working. The first is a recognition of the core expertise of each profession and a core knowledge related to professional training and experience. Second, interdisciplinary teamwork involves skill blending of common core skills between the different professions, which will enable a team to act as an integrated whole. Furthermore, many researchers, who espouse different methodologies, see collaboration as a key characteristic of research. Oja and Smelyan, for instance, state:

> The key characteristic of action research past and present is collaboration, which allows for mutual understanding and consensus, democratic decision making, and common action. (1989: 12)

Bines, Swain and Kaye present a similar rationale for teamwork in research:

> One of our strongest methodological reasons for our working as a team is centred on the potential value of bringing researchers with different perspectives and experiences together to both complement and correct the inevitable partialities of perspective and theory characteristic of any researcher. (1998: 75)

Research can not only require interdisciplinary teamwork, it can be the vehicle through which such collaboration is developed. Nevertheless, no matter how much diverse expertise is represented within the team, it will be of limited use unless it can be pooled. For this to happen, the group need to communicate effectively and openly.

Stop and Think
So, what are the potential difficulties? Make a list of the barriers to effective teamwork that might be found in collaborative research. (Hint: a good starting point is the general barriers to effective interdisciplinary teamwork.)

There are many potential barriers which you may have been able to list drawing on personal experience. Our list would include the following:

1. Perhaps the first set of barriers are those which prevent, distort or divert effective communication between the different members of the team. The effectiveness of interdisciplinary research depends on the personal qualities and skills of individuals, including motivation, confidence in their own professional roles and supportive working relationships.
2. There can be barriers in the operational and structural context, such as: the size of the team; the working base; the effectiveness of the formal channels of communication; the role of the 'leader' or co-ordinator; and the equality of working relationships. With regard to the last of these, Hilton concluded that, 'the research process will fail if one professional adopts an authoritarian approach' (1995: 36).
3. A third set of barriers emanates from professional boundaries, roles, expectations and lack of flexibility. Pietroni (1994), for instance, examined the ways in which stereotypes of each profession are established early on in professional careers and how expectations may affect communications and working relationships among staff from different disciplines.

Clearly the process of working with others is something to be worked on to realize the benefits of interdisciplinary research. Turning first to qualities and skills of effective individual team members, commonly recognized characteristics include: open-mindedness or the willingness to accept differences and the perspectives of others; negotiation skills; and willingness to accept new values, attitudes, and perceptions as appropriate.

French (1999) points out that effective teamwork cannot generally be left to chance in the process of working together. There are certain strategies and ways of working which promote effective working together. She cites four facets from Pritchard and Pritchard (1992):

1. Team members need to understand the goals of the team and the tasks they will perform as individuals. Thus it is vital that the team is working towards shared aims in the research project and can adopt the same strategies. In research using interviews, for instance, all those involved as interviewers will need to adopt the same interview protocol.
2. Teams work most effectively if members understand and value one another's roles. There needs to be appropriate assignment of tasks based on their skills. As Jenkins *et al* point out, 'when the team consists of members from different disciplines, the areas of expertise and the appropriate roles may be immediately evident' (1998: 62). Memberships and member roles may, however, need to remain fluid. Sometimes team members' expertise does not become fully apparent until later stages of the research.
3. Agreed procedures for carrying out tasks and evaluating them need to be negotiated.
4. Teams work most effectively if interpersonal relationships are good. Unresolved conflicts are likely to threaten seriously the effectiveness of the team (French, 1999: 261–262).

Furthermore, the problems that arise in working together can themselves be seen as productive rather than destructive. Jenkins *et al* (1998) suggest that disagreements and conflicts are inevitable, and learning to manage conflict is necessary for effective teamwork in research. Effective negotiation processes involve four main aspects (Thompson, 1996):

1. Separate the people from the problem.
2. Focus on interests, not positions. It is important that

members of the team are facilitated in expressing their interests. Individuals' interests need to be acknowledged as legitimate.

3. Generate possible options to further mutual interests. This involves a form of brainstorming in which the shared task is to produce a number of possible options for moving forward in a way that will be acceptable to all concerned.

4. Agree criteria for evaluating results.

In terms of the day-to-day business of working together, Jenkins *et al* (1998: 71–79) offer some time management strategies that may be used by the researching therapist. They suggest that effective time management is the result of planning so that the time available is used productively, and the most important strategy for time management is to include regular time to plan. When both long-term and specific short-term goals have been identified, planning can be devoted to action lists. It is important too to have regular research meetings: 'meetings with supervisors and colleagues are one of the activities that should be scheduled regularly to keep the project moving purposefully towards completion' (Jenkins *et al*, 1998: 74).

A major consideration in collaborative projects is that of co-authorship of publications. As Tripp-Reimer *et al* state:

> With regard to publications and presentations, it is advisable to establish at least preliminary guidelines during the formative stages of collaboration. Although these guidelines must remain somewhat flexible (depending on changing composition and contribution of team members), they serve to decrease fears and conflicts regarding credit for research effort. (1994: 329)

The issues of determining authorship for publications and presentations is of considerable importance as publications can be important for career enhancement. Clearly it is necessary that collaborators are given appropriate credit, but also that authorship is not credited when it is not earned. Tripp-Reimer *et al* suggest three general conditions for authorship credit, all of which must be met: substantial contributions to conceptualization and design of the study, or analysis and interpretation of data; drafting the paper or revising it critically for important intellectual content; and review and approval of the final version for publication (1998: 128).

As with any collaboration, there are different ways of organizing and working together. We have co-authored in three main ways. The first, and perhaps most obvious, is to divide the publication into sections and each of the co-authors takes responsibility for the first draft of an allotted section. This clearly relies on fairly substantial preplanning of the structure and content of the publication. For the second draft, the authors can either work on the same or different sections. A second way of organizing co-authorship, particularly in larger scale projects, is for each author to take the lead on different papers (or different publications). Thus if there are three authors, three papers are written each being credited to all three authors, the lead author being the first named. Again some preplanning is necessary to decide on the focus for each of the papers. The third way involves one author putting down some initial ideas. The second author modifies and extends this and then either passes it back to the first author or on to a third. Whichever way of organizing the collaboration is adopted, however, the key to writing together is the sharing and exchange of ideas and being able to comment on each other's work to facilitate each other's writing. Needless to say, there can be difficulties. It is not always easy to have your writing commented on by others. The four facets of effective teamwork outlined above are crucial to co-authorship.

Conclusion

Research tends to be seen as an individual rather than group or collaborative activity. This is, in part, a reflection of the association between research and the attainment of academic qualifications. PhDs, for instance, are not awarded to interdisciplinary teams and the thesis must be 'all your own work', whatever the degree of collaboration within the research. Nevertheless, research can be an effective vehicle for collaboration in which participants work together on all phases of a project which provides mutual benefits. Working with others, whatever your circumstances, should be integral to the research process whether this is with your supervisor, colleagues or other experts. It can be argued that a support network is essential for anyone who is embarking on a first research journey.

6

Literature review

Isaac Newton was one of the world's most original thinkers and scientists. Yet he expressed a certain humility about his achievements, explaining: ... 'If I have seen farther than others, it is because I was standing on the shoulders of giants' (see Thrower, 1990). It is in this spirit that researchers carry out a literature review – to ensure that their enquiry builds on the relevant work previously carried out by others. The literature review has five main functions for the researcher:

1. To help you understand the topic area thoroughly, through familiarizing yourself with the relevant previous theory and evidence.
2. To locate relevant methods (including accepted research designs and assessment tools) that have been adopted in relevant studies, and which might be applied in the current research.
3. To reveal gaps, unresolved issues and debates in the literature which the current study may address.
4. To provide a rationale for the current study.
5. To provide comparative results and an interpretative framework for analysing the findings of the current study.

For the reader of a research study, the literature sets out the intellectual context of the research. Not all of the literature reviewed needs to be published research. Opinion pieces, case studies and theoretical papers may all be relevant. In some areas of enquiry (such as the outcomes of creative arts therapies), there may be relatively little published research. The literature review may instead concentrate on published case studies and articles discussing professional experience. As in all reviews, it will be important to discuss the validity and generalizability of the information available.

The process of drawing up a literature review can appear taxing in both practical and emotional terms. The researcher may battle with constant uncertainty that the field has been thoroughly searched and all of the relevant references located. It may be difficult to place a boundary around the field of enquiry. Furthermore, some of the located papers and books may not be readily available. At first, the researcher may feel like a poorly equipped explorer of a new underground cave system, unsure whether newly uncovered passages will lead to amazing discoveries or simply to time-wasting dead-ends. It is not unusual for the researcher to spend much effort locating publications which on close reading have limited relevance to the project. It is clear that the processes of literature review take time and cannot be rushed. A variety of skills need to be developed. Yet the review process can be extremely interesting and rewarding. A researcher with sufficient time and skills (whether pursuing a well-contained undergraduate project or a major, well-funded study) will reap considerable personal satisfaction at developing expertise in the field, and becoming immersed in the research findings, methods and debates relating to the chosen area of enquiry. The purpose of this chapter is to introduce you to some key skills for carrying out this task.

As indicated in Chapter 4, the research process is often presented in linear form, starting with the literature review, and then moving on to the formulation of the research question, design of the method, and so on. This portrayal of the research process is rather simplistic. Whilst it is important to have a good knowledge of the literature at the project proposal stage, it remains important for researchers to stay abreast of the published literature throughout the project. Researchers who uncover unexpected findings (particularly likely in qualitative research) will certainly need to return to the research literature when analysing and discussing their results, in case there is another related field of enquiry that casts light on the findings. For example, Nochi (1998) interviewed people with traumatic brain injuries about their subjective experience of identity loss or change. In order to interpret participants' accounts more fully, the author reviewed further relevant work on labelling and social stigma in the discussion section of the paper.

Nevertheless, it is important for the researcher to place a boundary around the literature search. You may be interested in 'coping' issues, for example, but you will certainly not be able to read the 30,000 or so articles published in this field. You will need to focus on the evidence which directly addresses your research issue. You should also present your criteria for determining 'relevance' when writing the literature review.

The major processes of literature review

There are three major processes through which a literature review is created, and each process requires a number of specific skills:

1. Search and location of relevant literature.
2. Analysis and critical evaluation of individual sources of literature.
3. Synthesis – comparing, contrasting, organizing and presenting the written review.

As with all major intellectual tasks, the processes are not strictly sequential. For example, after critically evaluating a research study or methodology, the researcher may feel that it is necessary to go back to the search process again. For example, if the researcher has perceived some limitations to quantitative methods for measuring 'coping with chronic illness', previous qualitative research in this area may be more carefully searched. Even in the final writing up or 'synthesis' stage, certain conclusions may need to be checked by a final return to the literature. For example, if you reviewed the literature on depression in chronic illness, you might draw the conclusion that previous research has largely ignored ethnic and cultural differences in people's experiences. You might consider it prudent to search the literature once again in a very focused way to check that this statement is really justified.

Search and location of relevant literature

The search process usually moves from relatively general (e.g. all studies about coping with multiple sclerosis) to more specific, as the research question is gradually identified and sharpened (e.g. do people with multiple sclerosis who are depressed have differing levels of social support, or mobility problems, or reported fatigue, compared with those who are not depressed?). The literature search strategy may initially be relatively opportunistic, uncovering evidence that is readily available, in textbooks and in the professional journals that are at hand. Whether the researcher goes through this initial stage or not, all literature searches in the end need to become well directed and focused, or the researcher will almost certainly miss some of the necessary background information.

A decision will need to be made regarding inclusion or exclusion of papers published in other languages. Many researchers do not have the resources to seek translation. Nevertheless, some therapeutic techniques (such as the Feldenkrais method for working with posture and movement patterns) have been developed and studied mainly outside the UK and US. A review based on English language papers would in such cases be partial and potentially misleading.

Paper-based or traditional search approaches: The process of searching for relevant literature, which will provide the study's 'backdrop' of theory, methods and previous evidence, has been transformed by the development of electronic databases, and all researchers need to develop skills for searching these databases efficiently. Before looking at electronic search processes in more detail, we will consider the older, more 'traditional' methods of uncovering relevant information.

- Recommended, available books and articles and their references (e.g. textbooks, seminar materials, course reading lists).
- Review articles (and their references).

- Other experts, including charities and support organizations for disabled people.
- Manual search (scan through relevant sections within a university or medical library and the contents pages of current library stock journals that address the field of enquiry).

These methods can be helpful in the initial stages for determining a research area of personal interest and for formulating possible research questions. Review articles are especially useful for their extensive lists of references. However, do note that you are reading the reviewer's 'digest' of the articles and you may not come to the same conclusions if you read the original articles. It is intellectually safest to read the primary (original) sources of evidence, rather than relying on other people's reviews. Nevertheless, research reviews can provide a good entry point, and are particularly likely to be used to cover the older research on a topic. Then the researcher (especially one with limited time and resources) can focus on uncovering and analysing more recently published relevant research articles. For this, the electronic databases have become indispensable.

Electronic search: There are several electronic databases relevant to therapists, including Medline, CINAHL and PsycINFO. You may also gain access to the Cochrane database of systematic reviews. These examine available evidence for the effectiveness of specified treatments. You will need a user name and password, usually to be obtained through your library. You may then be able to access the databases from a home computer connected to the Internet, or alternatively you will be able to gain access through library terminals.

Each database provides many thousands of citations, and in most cases, the abstracts of research papers and books. Some articles (including Cochrane reviews) are available in 'full text' which can be printed out or downloaded on to disc. These are particularly valuable sources of information in the earlier stages of becoming familiar with a research area, and additionally supplement the search process by providing the references of all literature cited within the article itself. It is important to recognize that each database gathers material from somewhat different collections of journals and books. For example, Health Education Research (which may be important if you are examining an issue connected with health promotion or patients' responses to information) is not included in Medline, but is included in CINAHL and PsycINFO. Some journals that contain material relevant to research by therapists are not reviewed by any of these three databases (e.g. British Journal of Therapy & Rehabilitation, presently) and require a manual search approach. You can check if a journal that is of interest to you is included within a database by pressing the button 'Journal' at the top of the main search page (of each database) and then typing in and entering the journal title. Chalmers & Altman (1995) observe that a Medline search of treatment trials is unlikely to yield all published studies. However, the better quality trials are the ones most likely to be included within this database.

The basic search process is via 'keywords'. You type in a word relevant to your research topic and then click the mouse. The database will let you know how many articles have been found and then you can scan through their titles (and if relevant) their abstracts. The full text will be available in some cases. The titles are given in reverse chronological order, so that the most recent research is cited first. This 'basic' approach has two main drawbacks. Firstly, your 'keyword' may not align itself exactly with the database's preferred terminology. Secondly, a single keyword may return far too many citations to scan through. For example, 'coping behaviour' on Medline (1966–present) maps on to 'Adaptation, Psychological' and yields about 30,000 references.

Firstly, deal with the issue of keywords by exploring the terminology associated with your field. Many research articles (for example in the British Journal of Occupational Therapy) specify 'keywords'. You also need to explore the database itself. As indicated above, in Medline, the term 'coping behaviour' maps on to 'Adaptation, Psychological', and further terms. Enter different, but related words or phrases, and determine whether you are locating the same set or different articles. Be aware that you will uncover somewhat different sets of references depending on whether you enter the American or English spelling. In PsycINFO, the term 'coping behavior' yields more than 12,000 references, but 'coping behaviour' yields about a hundred.

A more advanced search strategy requires the use of further options, mostly provided by buttons along the top of the search page. The following suggestions do not exhaust the search opportunities and further possibilities will become apparent if you practise with the systems. You should also seek up-to-date training from your librarian.

Combine

If you enter two keywords, you gain two sets of references. For example, a key word 'Rheumatoid arthritis' will deliver all references containing this term within the database. Similarly, another key-word 'depression' will return all references relating to this particular term. A huge number of articles may appear in each set. If the button 'Combine' is then clicked (followed by clicking on each of the two sets) the result represents the intersection between the two original sets, and contains only articles that refer to *both* rheumatoid arthritis *and* depression. Further limitations can be placed by combining three or more sets (e.g. combining the above search with 'Women' to restrict the search to articles examining some aspect of rheumatoid arthritis, depression and women). The key challenge is to focus the search adequately – but not so much that important publications are missed. Another means of focusing is through the options AND/OR. For example, the keyword 'Exercise' in Medline results in two choices, 'Physiological' and 'Psychological'. By ticking both options and OR, you will be presented with information about all articles referring to exercise, whether the focus is physiology or psychology or both aspects. This is clearly a huge field of research and more than 5000 articles will be found. This is far too many for a researcher to scan through. If you select the AND button, you will be presented only with the articles that include reference to *both* the physiology *and* psychology of exercise. Articles referring to only one of these facets of well-being will not appear. This clearly reduces the field considerably. A researcher who is interested exclusively in psychological responses to exercise, would only select the option 'Psychological'. This operation would uncover several hundred references. A skilled researcher may attempt to focus the searched field even more narrowly, through the use of further keywords and the 'Combine' option. For example 'exercise (psychological)' and 'elderly' could be combined. Keep an accurate record of your search path through the keywords and options, as you may need to review these choices later and will probably have to outline your search strategy in the written review.

Limit

You may choose to limit the search (especially initially) for example, to topic reviews, article reviews or full text articles. This approach can yield detailed information at the earlier stages, perhaps leaving your search for specific research studies until later in the process when you are more focused and directed.

Author

This button is useful for searching for all work published by a given author. Alternatively, you can click your mouse on the cited authors when examining a title/abstract. For example, if you search for rheumatoid arthritis and pain, you may notice that Laurence Bradley has published in this field. If you click on the author's name, you will find dozens of studies that the author has published on pain. This may be very helpful for locating assessment tools and key concepts or models.

Journal

This button enables you to specify a journal – perhaps one that you have ready access to, so that you can read any cited articles quickly. This is especially useful when carrying out a preliminary search for a project proposal.

Change database

For topics that straddle medical/health and psychological research, you can run the same search using a different database – for example, moving from Medline or CINAHL to PsycINFO.

Stop and Think

Use Medline (date: 1966 to present) to search for articles on the effects of physical activity on falls among elderly people.

Hint: Use the following *Keywords*: Exercise, Falls.
These map to additional terms which you select (by clicking the mouse on them):

For 'Exercise': select physiology *or* psychology (to reach *all* articles on either topic). About 10,000 articles will be cited by the database.
For 'Falls': select option 'Accidental Falls', then further options 'Prevention/control' and 'mortality'. Nearly 1000 articles will be cited.

Combine the sets, using the appropriate button at the top of the main search page. The intersection of 'exercise' and 'falls' will provide a small number of references, including articles that perhaps you could locate immediately in your academic/medical library
Limit: Go back to 'Falls' and try '*Limit*' to 'topic reviews'. This time you will find more than 20 citations, reviewing litera-ture on treatment and prevention approaches. Again, a manageable set has been discovered, of great value in the early stages of conducting a search.

Locating relevant articles/books: Once you have enough references, the search process then moves on to locating the selected arti-cles and books. Clearly the local academic/medical library is the first place to look. However, no library can hold all the journals relevant to the health and social sciences. You may need to go further afield. It is often possible for researchers to gain inter-library loans through their own library. However, charges for this service are variable and can be quite high. A cheaper alternative may be to travel to other libraries which hold the rel-evant journals that you are seeking. You can find out which library you need, either by directly searching nearby university library catalogues through the Internet, or by using the Telnet service. Using Telnet, you type in the journal that you need and you will be given the names of libraries that hold that journal. There is a special service covering the large number of academic/medical libraries within the M25 (London) area. Do check the 'holdings' though, as many libraries do not hold the full set of journals from start to the present. Your library may be able to help you with this. It is recommended that you ring the library ahead of your planned visit to check on access policies and charges (if any).

Another option is to use the information resource centres of the College of Occupational Therapists, Chartered Society of Physiotherapy or the Royal College of Nursing. For some topics, specialist information can be accessed through charitable organizations such as the RNIB (Royal National Institute for the Blind) and RADAR (Royal Association for Disability and Rehabilitation). Their web-sites offer a useful introduction to their resources and services.

Throughout the search and review process, make sure to avoid bias in selecting publications. Resist the temptation to omit studies that challenge your point of view or research hypothesis! Contradictions within the literature need to be explored openly within the review. If the reviewer has been haphazard or selective in the literature surveyed, the review's conclusions cannot be considered valid or trustworthy (Chalmers & Altman, 1995).

It is really important to retain the complete details of all references read. This includes author, initials, title of paper, title of journal, volume and issue number, page numbers, and publishers of books. Records may be kept alongside your notes, or on cards. There are also electronic databases designed to keep track of references. A reliable form of organization will be invaluable. Many hours have been wasted by researchers who discover at the point of writing up their research, that they have mislaid the authors' initials, the page numbers of articles or similar seemingly trivial details!

Analysis and critical evaluation of individual sources of literature

Locating the relevant articles is only the first of the major literature review processes. The second process requires you to read each article carefully, analyse the key points, and critically evaluate the information. Indeed, you may need to read individual articles more than once, as you refine your argument and focus of enquiry.

There are two principal methods of recording the information that you extract from articles:

1. Summary notes: condensed records of each study, including the research question, main methods, sampling strategy, reliability/validity information, key findings, authors' interpretations and key limitations of the study.
2. Matrix or checklist approach: columns in which you summarize the research under similar headings.

Further notes should be kept, perhaps in a research log-book or journal, of the themes that you consider to be emerging from the literature. These will be useful later in the synthesis stage.

In order to read and critique a research article, you will need to apply your knowledge of research methods and statistics. You will also need to clarify the theoretical model that underpins the enquiry, think clearly about appropriateness of the design of the study, and examine the reliability and validity of the data collection methods. Do not be fearful of tables and graphs. Increasing familiarity with statistical concepts will help you to test at least their basic soundness. If means are compared, observe the standard deviations (SD) – if two groups are very different in the spread (SD) of scores, they may be drawn from very different populations, even if the means are similar. Consider the sample size and sampling strategy. If the sample is small, and 'volunteer' rather than randomly selected, is the researcher cautious about generalizing from the study? Compare results and discussion sections carefully as sometimes the author will misinterpret earlier tables or be over-ambitious in arguing the clinical significance of the findings. For example, correlational data may be interpreted over-confidently as suggesting cause and effect. Think about key limitations, both those that the researcher has admitted in the discussion section, and any that you have uncovered from your reading. For example, if you have read the article by Heck (1988), you will probably have queried why a logarithmic transformation of the data was justified, and you may have reservations about the implications that the author draws. Possibly you will also have queried whether variables that affect students' tolerance of brief electrical stimulation have relevance to patients who are coping with chronic pain.

Whilst it is important to approach research (and opinion papers) with informed scepticism, a certain humility is also recommended. It is rarely possible to design the 'perfect' study, especially with humans as participants. Even though a study may have flaws, it may nevertheless be useful, not least for suggesting issues and hypotheses that can be examined more thoroughly in subsequent work.

The 'analysis' stage entails detailed reconnoitring of the research 'landscape'. You may initially feel overwhelmed in detail and unable to 'see the wood for the trees'. Yet with time and immersion in the material, you will develop a detailed under-standing of the guiding theories, research methods, emerging philosophical assumptions, conflicting or puzzling findings, and the gaps in the evidence. When this occurs, you are ready to move into the synthesis stage.

Synthesis – comparing and contrasting studies, organizing the written review

The literature review that forms part of a project report or research article usually takes an 'essay' form. However, reviews may also include a table or matrix if many studies need to be summarized, accompanied by further discussion. There are also specialist statistical approaches to summarizing outcomes from a range of quantitative studies, such as meta-analysis, but these are beyond the scope of this chapter.

A poorly synthesized literature review tends to contain a simple listing of relevant studies, perhaps in chronological order of publication. Instead, careful attention needs to be given to the structure and presentation of the diverse material collected in the search and analysis stages. A variety of themes may have emerged from the literature, and thought needs to be given to their most logical ordering. There may be inconsistent defini-tions, diverse methodologies and contradictory research findings to explore. Subheadings may be helpful to map out the key themes or topic areas to the reader.

A literature review commonly has a 'funnel' shape, beginning with the more general issues or theoretical perspectives that form the background to the research, and then proceeds to examine more specific research studies that address the project's focus. Finally, the project's aims (questions or hypotheses) are presented and defended. A poor review often takes the form of a general essay that could be attached (loosely) to many different projects. Good reviews often have the following characteristics according to Chalmers & Altman (1995):

● They offer a summary of the process of literature search: the databases used, the keywords, and any criteria guiding inclusion or exclusion of studies. Where older reviews on the topic exist, they show how the current review is extending knowledge (what new research is included, or new perspectives).

● They highlight theoretical debates within the research area.

● They do not simply list relevant studies but they compare, contrast and evaluate their methods and results.

● As well as summarizing consistent patterns in previous research, contradictory findings are explored, and reasons (such as different measuring tools or sampling methods) are offered where possible.

● They reveal questions, gaps or contradictions in previous relevant literature, thereby providing a rationale for the proposed study.

● The style, structure, and level of detail will be appropriate for the intended audience (e.g. professional therapists, academic researchers, external examiner).

Brief reviews for research articles and project proposals will not display all of these qualities and will concentrate on establishing the most relevant previous research and its gaps and contradictions, so that the rationale for the current question or hypothesis becomes clear.

Stop and Think

Compare and contrast reviews

1. Examine the literature review section of a research article in a journal of your choice. Identify the basic plan of the review – how are the various relevant topics ordered and connected to the author's research question? Determine how many of the features suggested above are present within the review.

2. Read a systematic review, from the Cochrane collection. These are available in full text from the Biomed electronic database. Compare the content and presentation of the systematic review with the approach examined in (1).

Suggested articles

Britton, C. (1999) A pilot study exploring families' experience of caring for children with chronic arthritis: views from the inside. *British Journal of Occupational Therapy*, **62(12)**, 534–542.

Henry, K., Rosemond, C. & Eckert, L. (1999) Effect of number of home exercises on compliance and performance in adults over 65 years of age. *Physical Therapy*, **78(3)**, 270–277.

Van Tulder, M., Esmail, R., Bombardier, C. & Koes, B. (2000) Back schools for non-specific low back pain. *The Cochrane Database of Systematic Reviews*, **Issue (1)**.

Conclusion

The process of preparing an effective literature review requires time and several different academic skills. Particularly for those who are quite new to research, immersion in the relevant research literature will provide a vital 'apprenticeship' in the relevant theoretical models, methods and debates of the chosen field.

Sampling and sampling designs

Just a sample

A sample is a subset drawn from a given population. Argyrous provides a straightforward definition: 'a sample is a set of cases that does not include every member of the population' (2000: 4). Sampling in research has a number of associated key terms that will emerge as you progress through this chapter. 'Population' is one such term. The population may, for example, consist of all practising occupational therapists, and the sample will consist of a small number of them. The occupational therapists are, of course, drawn from a much wider population of therapists, employees, health workers, etc., and in that sense form a sample in themselves.

From the population of occupational therapists, a smaller group may be selected from which the actual sample is drawn; this is termed the 'sampling frame'. The occupational therapists in the sampling frame may, for example, work in a certain part of the country or in specific hospitals. In many areas of research which therapists conduct, it will be necessary to select individuals, hospitals, schools or pieces of text, from a wider population. We shall concentrate on sampling participants, which is the main concern in research for therapists, but we shall return to broader issues of sampling later in the chapter.

Stop and Think

Let us start with a fun example. Imagine you live in a large city. A friend is coming to visit and is bringing a very demanding colleague she wishes to impress. She wants to take him to the best restaurant in the city, and has listed a number of criteria for assessing restaurants; a wide selection of vegetarian food, swift service etc. So you have a research problem on your hands. Which restaurants will you visit for the purposes of this research? List a number of ways you might sample the restaurants to answer this research problem.

Maisel and Persell (1996) list seven general strategies for solving such sampling problems which provide a good basis for thinking about the issues involved.

1. *Census:* To conduct a census you would collect data by visiting every restaurant in the city. This approach may provide the best possible basis for answering your friend (as well as holding other attractions), but is likely, of course, to be well beyond your resources of time and money.
2. *Pseudo-census:* A pseudo-census is an attempt to visit as many restaurants as possible, though some will be missed (such as restaurants in public houses).
3. A *self-selected sample:* In this approach you would phone or e-mail all the restaurants, first explaining the problem and the criteria for assessing them, and then only visit those who respond positively.
4. A *convenience or haphazard sample:* You could visit a sample of convenient restaurants, in easy reach for you within the city.
5. A *typical case:* You might take the view that there is little difference between the restaurants of the type your friend is looking for and so just visit one typical example and send your friend the details.
6. A *quota sample:* Taking this strategy, you visit a cross-section

of restaurants in the city; for instance examples of restaurants in different areas of the city.

7. *A probability or random sample:* To do this you would need a full list of all the restaurants in the city. You then cut up the list, put all the names in a hat and pick out, say, ten to visit. This is a random sample.

This example may seem trivial, but we selected it for this very reason. Sampling can seem to be a highly technical procedure, but in an informal sense it is something we engage in as an everyday part of our lives. If you wish to buy car insurance, for instance, you might ring a sample of companies. We are constantly sampling in our everyday lives; we may, for example, look at several plants on display at the local garden centre and make the judgement that all the plants sold there are of a similar quality. We may sample the food in a newly opened restaurant and decide, after just one or two meals, that the cuisine or service is below standard. We could, of course, look at all the plants in the garden centre and try every item on the menu before making a decision, but it is unlikely that we would have the time, money or patience to do so.

Sampling as part of research is the same kind of process but differs in a number of ways:

- Sampling is approached more systematically in relation to the specific aims, purposes or hypothesis of the research. Sampling design is part of the decision-making process in research.
- There are practical considerations to be taken into account, such as the available time and resources.
- Perhaps above all, whatever approach or design you use in sampling in your research you need to be able to give reasons for doing it one way and not another. You need to be able to justify your approach.

In the remainder of this chapter we shall first explore some of the methodological issues involved in sampling, then outline some major approaches taken in research, and then look at some of the questions that arise in practice.

How sampling works in theory

The term 'sampling' originates within quantitative methodologies. It is a key statistical concept which generally refers to the selection of a group for research from a larger population so that the researcher will be able to make statements about the population as a whole. Most research in the area of therapy, as with all social research, involves search for, or at least consideration of, generalization. Essentially, the researcher is not primarily interested in the small group of people he or she has actually interviewed or observed for a limited time under specific conditions, but is wanting to treat the findings as typical of something wider, such as the effectiveness of a treatment for all patients with a given condition. Sampling a population is obviously more practicable and convenient than attempting to survey the entire population, and it also allows the researcher to obtain high quality information from just a few people. The question is, however: can the researcher make statements about everyone in the population based on the few that have been sampled? The extent to which the sample differs from the population it represents is termed the *sampling error*. This can never be eliminated completely, but it can be estimated statistically, allowing researchers to decide on the degree of error they are willing to accept. It is sometimes appropriate for researchers to discuss the sampling method they wish to use with a statistician.

Sampling is no less important in qualitative research. Selection underlies every phase of research, including selection of: the topic for investigation; methods of data collection and analysis; informants; time and places for observation; and what is observed and recorded. Within qualitative research, the whole notion of sampling has had, however, to be redefined. The search for systematic, intentional and theoretically guided approaches to sampling in qualitative research has seen the development of a number of strategies, including: purposive sampling; non-probability, which includes judgement, opportunistic and snowball sampling; and theoretical sampling (as discussed later in this chapter). Some qualitative researchers, however, explicitly claim not to intend generalizing their findings from their samplings. Questions of sampling are not simply technical issues. They address assumptions about the nature of the social world and whether it is desirable or even possible to make generalizations. If the social world is seen as rich in diversity and difference, ever changing and having meaning in specific historic and social contexts, then generalizations are deeply problematic. As Erlandson *et al* state: 'Rather than attempting to select isolated variables that are equivalent across contexts, the naturalistic researcher attempts to describe in great detail the interrelationships and intricacies of the context being studied' (1993: 32). Banister *et al* (1994) suggest that much qualitative research treats every study as if it were a single study, worthy of in-depth examination in its own right. Thus, there is no attempt to generalize beyond the specific case.

This is, however, one of those areas of contention in research. Silverman (2000) argues that generalizability can be desirable and possible in qualitative research. One possible strategy, he suggests, is to combine qualitative research with quantitative measures of populations. The simplest way of doing this is to compare your case study or findings, with the findings from other relevant case studies. It can be possible to discuss generalizability, in terms of similarities and differences to comparable cases, by reference to the literature. Certainly, as Carpenter and Hammell point out, in relation to therapy qualitative research, the plausibility of a study is partially evaluated through reference to systematic sampling:

> whether the method of sampling was relevant and appropriate; whether the sample relates to the group of which they are members; and whether a bias occurred due to either sampling or access. (2000: 111)

How to sample: probability sampling

The most basic distinction between sampling designs is between probability and non-probability designs. From the research practice point of view, probability designs involve randomization at some point in the process, whereas the generation of non-probability samples does not. Probability design can be a highly technical business related to statistical analysis (Argyrous, 2000).

Simple random sampling

A simple random sample is one in which every member of the population has an equal chance of being included. An example given by McCall (1996) is the measurement of the average resting heart rate of the population of the United Kingdom. A sample needs to be selected, as it would be impossible to measure the heart rate of every citizen. The researcher would wish to be able to estimate accurately the average heart rate of the population of the United Kingdom on the basis of the average heart rate of a random sample. In other words, the sample could be 'representative' and the findings generalizable to the whole population.

In general this method of sampling involves the random selection of the required number of individuals from a list of the total population, or sampling frame. Every member of the sampling frame is allotted a number and then a random selection is made using random number tables or a computer. Clearly the selection of a random sample depends on having a full and up-to-date list of the population.

But there are several reasons why simple probability samples can rarely be obtained in therapy research.

Stop and Think
You are working within a multi-professional team in Birmingham and wish to know the average resting heart rate of people with diabetes mellitus in Britain. What problems might there be in obtaining a random sample?

The following are general difficulties of securing a simple random sample:

● It is unlikely that anyone has compiled a completely accurate list of people with diabetes.

- The sample can be widely scattered between settings and geographically. It would be wrong, for example, to assume that a sample selected for patients at diabetes clinics in and around Birmingham would be representative of the country as a whole.
- The actual sample that the researcher obtains may not be representative of the population even if random selection is attempted. There are several reasons for this, including refusal to participate, non-availability of participants and exclusion for medical reasons. The researcher can randomly select others to be involved to replace those lost from the sample. The problem with this is, however, that those who did not participate, or did not volunteer to participate, may differ systematically from participants in unknown ways (for example attitude, life style, or social class). The numbers of people selected who do not participate depend on a number of factors, including the type of contact (for example postal surveys often have a low response rate), the type of person recruited (for example stigmatized groups such as drug addicts tend to respond poorly), and the amount of time and effort required.

One of the problems with medical research is that the people selected are normally patients, rather than people with similar health problems who do not seek medical advice, who are often the majority. Furthermore, as Bowling (1997: 210) points out, 'entry criteria to clinical trials of treatments are often restricted to patients with less severe conditions or more likely to benefit from the new treatment; this makes the findings of questionable generalizability.'

Systematic random sampling

Systematic random sampling offers a less time-consuming and laborious method of randomly selecting a sample than simple random sampling. It involves the selection of every nth case drawn from a sampling frame at fixed intervals. For example, if you have a list of 100 patients' names from which you wish to sample 10, an easy way is to start from a randomly chosen point and take every tenth name. (If you begin with the 6th name, you take the 16th, 26th etc.) This method of sampling can lead to a more even spread of the sample across the list than simple random sampling.

Stratified random sampling

To draw up a stratified random sample, the elements of the population are divided into non-overlapping groups, or strata. Simple random samples are then drawn from each of these groups. This method assures that certain characteristics of the population are represented (for example males and females or patients under 50 years old and patients over 50 years old). There are, however, certain disadvantages. It requires the names of all members of the population; and it can be costly and time-consuming to stratify lists.

Multi-stage sampling

With multi-stage sampling, groups are randomly sampled first and then individual participants are randomly sampled from these groups. For example, if you wanted to carry out some research on a sample of people with learning difficulties living in local authority hostels, you could first randomly select a group of hostels and then randomly select a group of people with learning difficulties from within these hostels. You may then go on to select randomly a further sample of people who had been in a hostel for more than one year, and another who had been there for less than six months.

This design helps to keep studies manageable and cheap by concentrating participants in a few places. If clients with learning difficulties were selected by means of simple random sampling for example, researchers would find themselves travelling all over the country. It is for these reasons that this approach is very common in therapy research.

Cluster sampling

With cluster sampling people or objects are selected in groups rather than on an individual bias. For example, cluster sampling of a few physiotherapy practices, and then a few therapists within each practice, saves time and expense by concentrating participants in a few locations.

How to sample: non-probability sampling

With non-probability sampling designs the researcher's subjective judgement plays a part in the selection of the sample. These designs are generally cheaper and easier to use and may serve the needs of individual therapists very adequately, according to the nature of their projects. As Argyrous states: 'There is no inherent reason why probability sampling should be considered "better" than non-probability sampling. Each method is appropriate for different research questions, and sometimes a research question will be better addressed by choosing a non-probability sampling method' (2000: 234).

Convenience sampling

With this type of sampling, people or objects are selected purely for convenience; the method is thus far from random. The sample may consist of a cohort of physiotherapy students from a particular college, a class of disabled children from a specific school, or a ward of patients from a particular hospital. Researchers using convenience samples will not be able to generalize their findings, but this may be of no importance, according to the aims of their research.

Purposive sampling (judgemental sampling)

With purposive sampling, the sample is hand picked by the researcher. For example, if the researcher has carried out a large questionnaire study, where the participants were randomly selected, he or she may then choose to interview a sample of specific people who are considered best able to answer a particular research question or who represent most diverse backgrounds.

Patton states: 'The logic and power of purposive sampling lies in selecting information-rich cases for study in depth. Information-rich cases are those from which one can learn a great deal about issues of central importance to the purpose of the research, thus the term purposive sampling' (1990: 169). He offers a number of strategies including: sampling extreme or deviant cases, or special or unusual cases; maximum variation sampling, or sampling unique variations that have emerged in adapting to different conditions; and criterion sampling, or sampling all cases that meet a criterion, such as all the patients in a treatment facility identified as having learning difficulties.

Snowball sampling

A snowball sample, so-called as it builds like a snowball, is selected on the recommendation of other participants. Typically, the researcher contacts one or two people and once trust has been established, and the participants have a good knowledge of what the research is about and what it entails, the researcher asks the first participants to nominate or introduce her or him to another person whom it would be useful to interview. The second wave of participants is then asked to nominate further participants, and so on. This form of sampling may be most useful when a relatively hidden, sometimes deviant, group of participants is being sought. Domholdt (2000) gives the example of a study of patients who return to sporting activities earlier than recommended after ligament reconstruction surgery. If the researchers can use personal contacts to identify a few subjects, it is likely that those subjects will be able to identify other potential subjects.

Quota Sampling

Quota sampling is a widely used method of non-probability sampling. As for stratified sampling, the population is spilt up into non-overlapping sub-groups. Relevant sub-groups in therapy research might be specified according to age, sex, religion, ethnicity, medical diagnosis and socio-economic status. Thus, for instance, a researcher may interview 10 male patients and 10 female patients. Whilst stratified random sampling involves a random sampling method of selecting respondents, quota samples are selected on the basis of opportunity or convenience. In research in which the proportion of the different groups within the population is known, for example in research into colour blindness, which effects a proportionally higher number of males than females, this can be reflected in the quotas of males and females in the sample quotas. As Schofield states, however:

> The major problem with quota sampling is that attempts to deal with one known source of bias may well make matters worse for others not known, or at least not known until after the data is collected and it is too late. (1996: 36)

For example, if a study compared married and widowed quotas of old people coping with a certain health condition, we might find later that widowed status was associated with greater poverty, confusing our understanding of illness stress-coping issues.

Some questions arising in practice

Which sampling method should be used?

The appropriate sampling method will depend on your research questions and the resources and time available to you. It may be vital for you to generalize your findings but, alternatively, this may not be one of your aims. In research, compromises constantly have to be made; what you want to do may be different from what, in theoretical terms, it would be best for you to do. For example, you may ideally require a large random sample, but time and money constraints may only allow either a large convenience sample or a small random sample. In cases such as this, you will need to decide whether the size or the 'randomness' of the sample is the most important factor.

What size should the sample be?

A major decision that researchers must make when planning their research is the number of participants required for their sample. The problem has no simple or general answer and will depend upon a variety of factors. Sample size should be decided in advance, otherwise it may look as if you stopped collecting data as soon as your hypothesis was supported. With some research approaches and designs it is perfectly legitimate to have just one participant in your sample. In probability sample designs, however, sample size is more a matter of statistics, and formulae for calculating required sample size and sampling error can be found in statistics textbooks. In general, the following factors should be taken into consideration when deciding on the size of your sample.

Practical considerations: There are many practical considerations to be taken into account concerning the availability of partici-pants, and how much a large sample would cost to contact in terms of time and money. Therapy students carrying out small projects as part of their final year of study, for example, would be ill-advised to contemplate a sample of more than a few. As noted above, some sampling designs group participants together, which can be an enormous saving in terms of time and resources.

Representation and generalization: If a representative sample is important, the sample should be large enough to provide stable values; that is, another similarly chosen sample from the same population should not yield results that diverge appreciably from those obtained.

Variability of results: Another consideration which needs to be made when deciding on the sample size is the degree of variabil-ity in results that can be expected on the basis of previous expe-rience. For example, experiments involving the measurement of reaction time to a stimulus such as light require fewer partici-pants than experiments measuring complex motor skills or atti-tudes, because in the former case there is far less variability from one person to another. Variability is also affected by the homo-geneity of the sample; the more alike the individuals are, the less variability they will display and the smaller the sample need be.

Purpose of the research: The size of the sample will also depend on the purpose underlying the research. If it is a pilot study, where the purpose may be to smooth out any problems in the research design, then using a large sample would be wasteful and unnecessary. Similarly in undergraduate research the main purpose is to demonstrate to the examiners that basic research procedures have been tackled and that learning about the research process has taken place. In this situation a large sample would be neither sensible nor necessary.

Size of the population: If the size of the population under consideration is small, then a small sample may represent a large proportion of the population. If, for example, you wanted to research visually impaired physiotherapists who are currently practising in the United Kingdom, your total population would be no more than 250, so a sample of 50 would be considerable. If, on the other hand, you wanted to study female physiotherapists, where the population contains many thousands, a sample of 50 might be insufficient.

Type of participants: With any research project, participants are always lost. They may become uninterested and drop out, move, fail to turn up for interview, spoil their questionnaires or forget to send them back. It is possible for researchers who have had some experience to make reasonably accurate guesses as to the likelihood of this happening in their research. It might be expected, for example, that a sample of therapists, interested in the topic under investigation, might be more committed than a sample drawn at random from the public. If you suspect that a large number of participants will drop out of your study, or that they may be less than dependable, it is wise to start with a larger sample than you need.

Sampling for other reasons

The sampling designs described above apply to the selection of research participants. There are however other aspects of sampling that can be involved in research. Documentary research, for instance, can involve sampling (see Chapter 13). A content analysis of the last five years of a professional journal to find significant changes in the attitudes of therapists to physical illnesses might involve a sample of two editions each year. In observation studies, systematic sampling helps ensure that 'a representative sample of behaviours is obtained, that generalizations can be made from the observed sample to a wider sample and that a detailed understanding of the observed events is gained' (Seale and Barnard, 1998: 77) (see Chapter 12).

Conclusion

Sampling is a decision-making process in all therapy research. The sampling design and the size of the sample need careful consideration and will be affected by constraints of time and resources. Sampling decisions are crucial for researchers to justify the particular designs they adopt. The major factors include the realization of the aims of the research; time constraints; and available resources. Of these, the aims or purposes of your research will be of paramount importance. Sampling, particularly probability sampling, can be a technical business. As Argyrous states, however: 'the choice of research methods should never be undertaken on the basis of the technique to be used for analysing data. It should be chosen on the basis of best addressing the research problem at hand' (2000: 235).

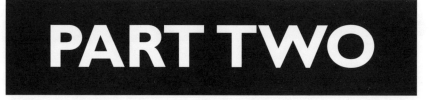

PART TWO

RESEARCH METHODS AND APPROACHES

8

The questionnaire

The questionnaire is a research tool where information is gathered about groups of individuals in a systematic way. A questionnaire simply consists of a list of questions, but its construction is quite an arduous task and one that needs considerable practice.

Questionnaires can be distributed to research participants in four main ways:

1. They may be delivered by post.
2. The researcher may deliver them personally, in which case groups of individuals may complete the questionnaire in one place and at one time.
3. The researcher may go through the questions verbally with each research participant. This is often referred to as a structured interview and will be considered in Chapter 9.
4. The researcher may send the questionnaires to a person in authority, for example a therapy manager, who will distribute them, collect them, and send them back to the researcher. It saves considerable postage if the questionnaires can be sent in bulk, especially as stamped addressed envelopes are required for their return.

As with all research methods, you need to be clear why you want to use the questionnaire. The questionnaire is very familiar to most people, and can reach a large number of people very easily; for these reasons there is a tendency to use it indiscriminately.

Before deciding whether the questionnaire is the best research tool, you need to have a clearly formulated research question and a definite idea of the kind of information you require. If you want to learn about people's deepest thoughts on a topic, for example, an unstructured or semi-structured interview would almost certainly be more suitable. You also need to consider who your sample will comprise; a questionnaire is unlikely to provide useful data from young children or from people who cannot read.

Even when you have made the decision to use a questionnaire, many other factors need to be considered before you can proceed with its design. You will need to decide on the sample size that you require, how you will distribute the questionnaire, how you will analyse the data, whether or not you need to consult a statistician, and whether it will be your only research tool. You may even find an existing questionnaire which suits your needs, or one that you can modify. Weerakoon and O'Sullivan (1998), in their study of inappropriate patient sexual behaviour in physiotherapy practice, modified an existing questionnaire which had itself been constructed from three other questionnaires. Many questionnaires exist to measure, for example, depression and functional independence. They can be useful in some research studies and may help to provide additional, validated data to compare with the data collected through your own questionnaires.

Types of questions

Questionnaire items can be divided into two basic types: closed questions which are structured in such a way that research participants' answers are constrained; and open questions which allow research participants to answer in their own words.

Closed questions

Dichotomous questions ('Yes/No'questions): With dichotomous questions the research participant is only permitted to answer 'yes' or 'no'. With some very factual questions this is all that is required. For example:

Were you over the age of 25 when you commenced your occupational therapy course?   Yes ....   No ....

With some 'Yes/No' questions it is wise to allow research participants to indicate that they do not know the answer. For example:

Did the number of patients with multiple sclerosis treated in your department exceed 50 last year?

Yes ....
No ....
Don't know ....

Johnson and Sim (1998) used dichotomous questions in their comparative study of the knowledge and attitudes of physiotherapy and occupational therapy students towards AIDS and HIV. Below is an example from their research:

All blood products used for transfusions in the UK are now screened for HIV.   Yes ....   No ....

Scaled questions: A scale represents a series of ordered steps or fixed intervals which are used as a standard of measurement. Scales provide numerical scores which can be used to compare individuals and groups. They are sometimes referred to as Likert scales, which were developed by Rensis Likert. With scaled questions, research participants are given a little more scope to express their views than they are with dichotomous questions, but their responses are still restrained. Scales usually comprise five points. An example may be:

I enjoy my current employment. Please circle the number that best expresses your view.

Strongly agree	Agree	Neither agree nor disagree	Disagree	Strongly disagree
1	2	3	4	5

Some researchers prefer 'strongly agree' to correspond to number 5 so that if the scores are added up across questions, high scores reflect positive attitudes.

Rather than labelling scales according to whether research participants agree or disagree, a particular concept, such as 'interest' or 'enjoyment', may be expressed throughout the scale. For example:

How interesting do you find anatomy? Please circle the number than best expresses your view.

Very interesting	Interesting	Neither interesting nor uninteresting	Uninteresting	Very uninteresting
1	2	3	4	5

The same idea must be expressed throughout the scale or great confusion will result. For example, it is no use starting the scale with 'very enjoyable' and ending it with 'very uninteresting'; although this sounds obvious, it is a mistake that is frequently made. The wording of the points on the scale also need attention; it is easy for research participants to discriminate between 'agree' and 'disagree', but if they are asked to discriminate between 'often' and 'frequently' their responses will be unreliable. Sometimes the scale is only labelled at either end.

Johnson and Sim (1998) used five point scales in their comparative study of the knowledge and attitudes of physiotherapy and occupational therapy students towards AIDS and HIV. Below is an example from their research:

I do not feel much sympathy for anyone who catches the virus through drug abuse.

Strongly Agree				Strongly disagree
1	2	3	4	5

Attitudes are very complex and it is usually necessary, when attempting to measure them, to present several scales relating to the same concept. For example, when attempting to measure job satisfaction, you may want to ask about pay, working conditions, promotion prospects, supervision, and sense of achievement. One problem with the analysis of scales, is that research participants can have identical overall scores but arrive at them in different ways. Some may, for example, be dissatisfied with their pay and conditions, some with the nature of the work itself, and others with their managers. Researchers are, of course, free to study the responses of individual research respondents or specific items on the questionnaire if they wish.

Providing several scales on a topic, rather than one global question, may also help to minimize the 'halo effect'. The 'halo effect' refers to the tendency we have to view everything about a person we like as 'good' and everything about a person we dislike as 'bad'. Thus rather than asking clinical tutors 'How well did this student perform in your department?', it would be best to break the question down into various aspects concerned with communication, assessment, clinical interviewing, punctuality and so on.

Scaled questions can have more than five points, but if there are more than seven, research participants tend to find discrimination difficult. Some researchers prefer to keep the number of points on the scale even, for example four points rather than five. This is because the middle point of the scale can be difficult to interpret, especially if the scale is only labelled at either end. Circling the middle point of the scale may mean that research participants have no opinion on the topic, that they do not know the answer, or that they do not want to think about the question. If there are four points on the scale research participants are forced to come down on one side or the other, but they may become irritated by this. Having no middle point can also distort the data if research participants' attitudes genuinely lie at the centre.

A further problem with scales is that research participants are inclined to circle the same number consistently; this tendency is referred to as 'response set'. As noted above, this frequently occurs with the middle point of the scale. The extremes of the scale, on the other hand, tend to be avoided. Some researchers have advocated alternating the direction of the scales as a way of reducing 'response set'. Thus on some scales 'Strongly agree' could be placed on the left hand side, and on others it could be placed on the right hand side. This procedure does, however, tend to be confusing, as well as making the analysis more difficult for the researcher. Using other types of questions to break up a list of scaled items may also help to reduce 'response set'.

Tick lists: Another method of eliciting closed answers is to ask research participants to tick items from a list. For example:

In your view which of the following treatment modalities are effective in relieving the pain of frozen shoulder? Please tick as many items on the list as you wish.

1. Ice
2. Infra-red irradiation
3. Ultra-sound
4. Short-wave diathermy
5. Exercise
7. Manipulation

When presenting a list such as this, it is wise to include an 'other' category. This having been said, research participants do not use this category very readily as they find it much easier to recognize items from a list than to bring them to mind. It is important, therefore, that your list is as exhaustive as possible. You may wish to limit research participants to a certain number of responses; with the above example, for instance, you could ask them to tick the three modalities which they believe to be most effective in relieving the pain of frozen shoulder.

You may also ask research participants to place themselves in categories. For example:

Please indicate to which age group you belong.

18–28	....
29–38	....
39–48	....
49–58	....
59 or over	....

It is important to ensure that categories do not overlap. This is a common error when categorizing age groups and can cause great confusion. For example:

18-28   ....
28-38   ....
38-49   ....

In this case it would be difficult to categorize a person aged 28 or 38.

Research participants may also be asked to indicate an amount. For example:

Please indicate how many patients you treated today?

0– 5   ....
6–10   ....
11–15   ....
16–20   ....
20 or over ....

Weerakoon and O'Sullivan (1998), in their study of inappropriate patient sexual behaviour in physiotherapy practice, asked research respondents to tick one of four alternatives to a series of questions. An example from their research is given below:

Were you ever in a situation where a patient asked you for a date?

Never   ....
Once   ....
More than once with the same individual   ....
More than once with different individuals   ....

Ranking: Another type of closed question is where research participants are asked to rank items on a list. For example, if you were carrying out a study to ascertain the popularity of various items on sale in the hospital canteen, you might devise the following question:

Please rank in order of preference the following desserts on sale in the hospital canteen. Give the item you most prefer number 1 and the item you least prefer number 8.

Bread pudding   ....
Fruit salad   ....
Rice pudding   ....
Yoghurt   ....
Apple pie   ....
Jelly   ....
Ice-cream   ....
Steamed pudding ....

The word 'prefer' would, however, be rather confusing as some research participants might love bread pudding but avoid it for fear of gaining weight or in the interests of eating a 'healthy' diet. This illustrates the importance of knowing exactly what information you require and of avoiding ambiguity.

Multiple-choice questions: Closed questions can also test research participants' knowledge in a multiple-choice format. It is essential that there is only one correct answer. For example:

The normal pH of the blood is:

1.   7.2   ....
2.   7.6   ....
3.   7.8   ....
4.   7.4   ....

It is desirable when constructing multiple choice questions, that each alternative is approximately the same length, as research participants have a tendency to choose the 'odd one out'.

Matrix questions (grid questions): If you want to ask two or more questions at once a grid can be used. In the following example the researcher wants to know how long a sample of physiotherapists have worked in a variety of specialities since they qualified. Research participants would be asked to place a tick in the appropriate boxes.

How long have you spent in each of these specialties since qualifying?

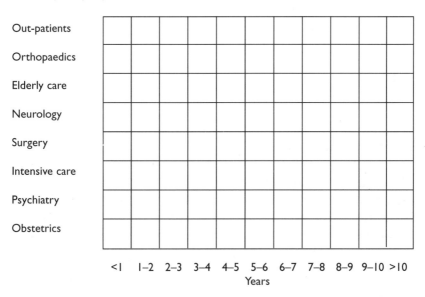

Figure 8.1 Matrix question

Stop and Think
Think of a simple research question, for example people's motives for becoming physiotherapists or occupational therapists, and devise a questionnaire using some of the closed question types described above. Try the questionnaire out on a friend to check that all the questions are clear.

Open questions

Open questions allow research participants to answer in their own words, the only real restraint being the amount of space provided on the questionnaire. An example might be:

Please explain why you find it difficult to come for physiotherapy treatment regularly.

Questionnaires usually have a mixture of open and closed questions. After circling a point on a scale, for example, research participants may be asked to explain their view. It is also common for questionnaires to end with an open item such as:

Please give any other information that you feel is important.

Open questions can provide a wealth of rich information, but they are more time-consuming than closed questions to respond to and analyse. In addition research participants may find it arduous to express themselves in writing, or be unprepared to give the task their time. If you find you need to ask a lot of open questions, you should seriously consider whether the interview would be more appropriate. Researchers frequently conduct some interviews as well as using questionnaires in order to gain depth as well as breadth of knowledge. Jepson (1998), for example, in her study of the equipment needs of people with restricted growth, sent 90 questionnaires and carried out ten interviews.

Stop and Think

Return to the above activity where you devised a short questionnaire using closed questions. Add two or three open questions to your questionnaire. Write a paragraph explaining how this is likely to change the information you have gathered.

Filter questions

Filter questions are used to indicate whether or not the questions that follow are relevant to the research participant. If they are not, the research participant is directed to miss them out and proceed to another question or section of the questionnaire. An example of a filter question might be:

Did you qualify as an occupational therapist before 1980?

Yes ....   No ....

(If your answer to this question is 'No' please proceed to section B.)

Funnel questions

Funnel questions seek more and more detailed information on one particular topic. They were used by Britton (1999) in her study of the experiences of families who care for children with chronic arthritis. An example from this research is given below:

How long was there between the first signs of illness and the child being given a firm diagnosis?

Do you think the time taken between first illness and diagnosis made any difference to how you coped later?

Can you say how it made a difference?

The use of pictures

Pictures or photographs can be used in questionnaires. For example, in a study to ascertain children's knowledge of back care and lifting, the therapist could present the children with pictures of 'stick people' lifting objects in various positions, and ask them to indicate which they consider 'good' and which they consider 'bad'. Similarly the points on a scale could be presented in pictorial form, like the one in Figure 8.2 overleaf.

The wording of questions

The wording of questions on a questionnaire is vitally important and needs a great deal of care. Judd *et al* (1991) note that even small changes in wording can bring about large changes in response.

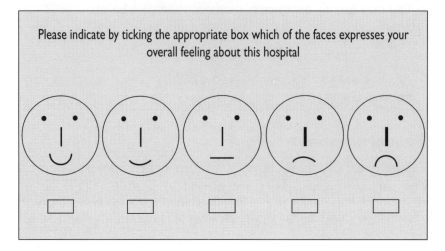

Please indicate by ticking the appropriate box which of the faces expresses your overall feeling about this hospital

Figure 8.2 Pictorial questions

Below are listed some particular types of questions to avoid. This should be viewed merely as a guide; it can be difficult to circumvent all the problems mentioned all of the time.

Leading questions

Leading questions influence the direction of research participants' replies by indicating the way in which the researcher wants them to answer. An example might be:

> Please indicate how you feel about the splendid new hydrotherapy pool.

The word 'splendid' indicates to research participants that the researcher expects them to be pleased with the hydrotherapy pool.

Even if a scale is provided where shades of opinion can be expressed, the question may still be leading. For example:

> Indicate how much improvement has taken place in your pain over the last month. Please circle the point on the scale that best expresses your view.

Very much improved	Improved	No different	Is worse	Is very much worse
1	2	3	4	5

By mentioning 'improvement' in the question, the research participant is given the message that this is what is expected, and that this is what the researcher wants to hear. Avoiding leading questions such as this is not always easy, though the words 'if any' after 'improvement' would make the question more neutral. One way round the problem of leading questions is to word some questions positively and other questions negatively; for example some could mention 'improvement' while others could mention 'deterioration'. This, however, tends to be confusing to research participants, and to researchers when they come to analyse the data.

Leading questions can occasionally be used to advantage if the information sought involves behaviour which is socially disapproved of, leading to denial, as they have the effect of indicating to research participants that such behaviour is 'normal' and expected by researchers and that they will be tolerant of it. For example rather than asking:

How you taken any time off work because of your backache?

The researcher could ask:

How much time have you taken off work because of your backache?

There is an ethical issue in using leading questions in this way as researchers are extracting information from research participants which, under ordinary circumstances, they may not be prepared to give.

Loaded questions

A loaded question is one which suggests a judgement and is imbued with feelings of approval or disapproval. Questions, statements and response options which are coloured with moral judgements and evaluations should generally be avoided, otherwise the research participant is likely to react to the emotional, rather than the factual, content of the question. Emotive words such as 'justice' and 'equality' should generally be avoided, as well as any word or phrase which implies the researcher's values or which could be offensive to the research participants. It is not always easy to avoid loaded questions, however, because what is regarded as judgemental by one person may be viewed as neutral by another.

People have a tendency to present themselves in the best possible light to others; this has been termed the 'social desirability effect'. This tendency operates when people fill in questionnaires, even though the questionnaire is anonymous and they are unlikely to meet the researcher. In some questionnaires, for example Eysenk's Personality Questionnaire, a series of questions, often called a lie scale, are included as a way of detecting the social desirability effect. Such questions might include:

Have you ever been late for work?   Yes .... No ....
Have you ever been unkind to anyone? Yes .... No ....

Research participants who consistently say 'no' to items such as these, are believed to be susceptible to the social desirability effect and their scores can be adjusted to accommodate this.

A series of questions, rather than a single general question, can reduce the social desirability effect. For example, in response to the question 'Do you like children?', many research participants may feel they ought to say 'yes' because they believe that is what society expects of them. However, if a series of questions or statements concerning attitudes towards children are asked, rather than a single global question, a far more complex picture is likely to emerge.

Multiple questions (double-barrelled questions)

These questions require more than one response and are therefore difficult or impossible to answer correctly, especially if they are closed. An example might be:

Please indicate how much pain and stiffness you are now experiencing in your elbow.

A great deal ....
Some   ....
A little   ....
None   ....

These questions are highly perplexing to research participants and will create unreliable data. This is because they may want to say 'yes' to one half of the question and 'no' to the other half. Double-barrelled questions are also very confusing to researchers when they come to analyse the data.

Ambiguous questions

Ambiguous questions are ones which invite various interpretations; they need to be avoided, especially as there is no opportunity of clarifying their meaning as there might be in an interview. Very often the ambiguity centres around an ordinary word or phrase, for example 'frequently' or 'occasionally'. At other times the whole sentence may be ambiguous or confusing. For example:

Please indicate how many times you carried out the exercises last week.

The research participant may be left wondering whether the researcher means the number of times a group of exercises were carried out, or the number of times individual exercises were carried out.

Assuming questions

These questions make assumptions about research participants' lifestyles, behaviour or attitudes. For example, questionnaires on disability might assume that people who use wheelchairs want to walk. Similarly questions such as 'Do you have adequate study leave?' assumes that study leave is valued by research participants.

Irrelevant questions

It is tempting to include items on questionnaires merely to satisfy curiosity, or because the information *might* be important. Irrelevant questions should, however, be avoided: they make the questionnaire longer, which may lower the return rate, and they give research participants and researchers unnecessary work. In addition if an irrelevant question irritates or offends research participants, co-operation may be lost unnecessarily. Denscombe writes that:

> ... the researcher has to walk a tightrope between ensuring coverage of all the vital issues and ensuring that the questionnaire is brief enough to encourage people to bother answering it. (1998: 96)

Questions full of jargon

Questions full of jargon and abbreviations should be avoided unless you are sure research participants will understand their meanings.

Occupational jargon becomes so familiar to those 'in the know' that it is easy to include it unwittingly in questionnaire items. It is easy, for example, for occupational therapists to use 'OT' in questionnaires without realizing that some research respondents will not know the meaning of the abbreviation.

Questions phrased in the negative

Questions phrased in the negative take longer to process cognitively, and can give rise to confusion and incorrect answers if research participants are not fully concentrating. They are best avoided wherever possible. An example of a negatively phrased questionnaire item is:

> Please indicate how many times you did not do your exercises last week.

It is much less confusing to ask research participants how many times they *did* do their exercises. If negative words must be used they need to stand out in some way, for example by underlining them or by using bold print.

The sequence of questions

On most occasions it is best to begin the questionnaire by asking for factual information of a neutral kind. If you start with intimate or highly personal questions you may alienate the research participants. It should be noted, however, that even simple demographic questions are viewed by some research participants as intimate, for example questions asking for details of age or ethnic origin. It is important to hold the research participant's interest throughout the questionnaire, so some of the more interesting questions could be reserved until the end. It is probably best to place the more difficult or time-consuming questions in the middle of the questionnaire.

People like to appear consistent, so when ordering questions, it is important that their answers to one question do not influence their answers to the next. This can be difficult because it is disconcerting for research participants if questionnaires swing markedly from one topic to another.

Stop and Think
Construct a short questionnaire to investigate a topic that interests you. Use a mixture of open and closed questions. See how far you can avoid the pitfalls that have just been described.

Return rates

The return rate of questionnaires varies according to who the research participants are, but generally speaking it tends to be low (Denscombe, 1998). May (1997) gives a figure of 40% which may be even lower with a random sample of the general public. Return rates are higher if research participants complete the questionnaires under the direction of the researcher. Return rates of 60 or 70% are not unusual when questionnaires are sent to therapists. Beeston *et al* (1998), for example, in their study concerning the uptake of Master's degree programmes among physiotherapists, report a response rate of 89% for managers and 61% for clinicians. Postal questionnaire surveys, in particular, tend to yield disappointingly low returns.

If your response rate is unsatisfactory, you can send reminders to those who failed to respond; in order to do this it is necessary to identify each questionnaire with a number before it is sent. This, however, gives rise to an ethical dilemma regarding anonymity.

Even if your return rate is good, it may be worthwhile to pursue those who have failed to reply. People who fail to respond are rather different from those who do, and so by persuading them to co-operate your sample will be more representative. Reminders suffer from the law of 'diminishing returns', however, with each yielding less and less questionnaires.

As the response rate of questionnaires is typically low, everything needs to be done to persuade the research participants to respond. Researchers may increase the response rate by ensuring that questionnaires are easy to complete, attractive and 'user friendly'.

Stop and Think
Make a list of all the things you could do to tempt research participants to complete your questionnaire and thus to improve the response rate.

The following tips may help to improve the return rate:

- Use good quality paper. This is particularly important if the questionnaire is sent through the post.
- Use a clear font. A large font may also be needed by research respondents with visual impairments.
- Provide sufficient space for research participants to write their responses.

- Provide very clear instructions on how to answer the question at each new sub-section. Instructions should be put in bold print or a different font type from the rest of the text.
- Make sure response boxes are in correct alignment to the questions.
- Use a computer to construct the questionnaire rather than handwriting.
- Number the pages and indicate when pages should be turned.
- Enclose a stamped addressed envelope.
- Offer to send an abstract of the results to the research participant.
- Thank the research participant at the end of the questionnaire.
- Clearly specify the return date and do not make it too distant, two to three weeks is a reasonable time-span.
- Ensure confidentiality and anonymity if this is your intention.
- Enclose an explanatory letter which states who you are and the purpose of your study. It may help to name your sponsors (if any), your qualifications, and where you are studying or working. It is also important to tell research participants how they were selected. Write in a straightforward, courteous way, making your research sound interesting and worthwhile.
- Material incentives are sometimes offered to research participants which may improve return rates, but most researchers cannot afford them. It may also be regarded as coercive.
- Do not make the research participants work unnecessarily. Try to ensure that they complete the questionnaire at a time and in a place which is convenient to them. Avoid the height of any holiday season, such as Christmas, when sending out questionnaires as people tend to be very busy. Do not ask research participants for information they are unable to give, or which would be inconvenient for them to find. For example, it is probably unreasonable to ask a junior therapist questions about the departmental budget.
- Provide research participants with 'bridging statements' when topics change within the questionnaire as people tend

to find sudden changes of subject disconcerting. Short bridging statements such as 'The following section will ask for your opinions on clinical education', preceding each change of topic, will help to refocus research participants' attention.

● If filter questions are used it is very important to make sure research participants can find their way around the questionnaire without difficulty.

The pilot study

Before the questionnaires are printed in large numbers and distributed, it is important to test them on a few people to eliminate any remaining problems that may have been overlooked. However careful you may have been, a few trifling problems will usually remain; for example a question may be slightly ambiguous, or a space for an open response may be too small.

The people in the pilot study should be as similar to the 'real' research participants as possible. It is wise to encourage them to be critical, and to give their opinions on the length of the questionnaire, its clarity and attractiveness, any problems they encountered with specific questions, and any adverse reactions they had. If you have difficulty finding a sample of people to take part in your research, it is probably not worth 'wasting' them on the pilot study. In this situation it is legitimate to choose people who are dissimilar, yet as similar as possible, to the survey participants. Those who participate in the pilot study can, however, take part in the main study if it needs no modification. It may also be legitimate to include the participants of the pilot study if the main study is using participative research methods (see Chapter 17).

Analysing questionnaire data

Closed questions are amenable to a statistical analysis. To analyse data numerically or statistically using a computer, every item and sub-item on the questionnaire must be given a number.

You may choose to pre-code your questionnaire in this way; for example a list of items may be numbered, as may the five points on a five point scale. You may wish to display your data as graphs, tables, charts and simple statistics, for example means, modes and percentages (see Chapter 15). Open-ended questions can be analysed by means of content analysis and other qualitative methods (see Chapter 15).

Disadvantages of questionnaires

> **Stop and Think**
> What do you consider to be the main advantages and disadvantages of the questionnaire as a research tool? You may like to think about the questionnaires you constructed earlier to help answer this question.

When deciding which research method or methods to use, the researcher has much to consider, not least the many practical issues which inevitably arise. All other things being equal, however, the questionnaire can be said to have the following advantages and disadvantages:

Advantages
- It is relatively cheap in terms of time and money.
- A large number of individuals can be reached relatively easily and inexpensively.
- The lack of face-to-face contact between the researcher and the research participants reduces certain psychological and social influences, i.e. the questionnaire is a relatively non-reactive technique.
- Research participants have more time to think than they do in the interview, and can complete the questionnaire in their own time.
- The analysis of the data is relatively speedy.

Disadvantages

- The information gathered tends to be rather superficial as it imposes structure on the research participants' responses. This may, however, be of no concern according to the research question or aims.
- Lack of contact between the research participant and the researcher means that questions cannot be clarified or reworded.
- Unless questionnaires are pictorial, they are unsuitable for certain people, for example young children, and those who cannot read.
- The response rate tends to be poor and some questionnaires may be returned incomplete or poorly completed.

Conclusion

The questionnaire is a very popular and familiar research tool and one which is of immense use to researchers. A range of questions, from those which are highly structured to those which are totally open, can be devised to answer a huge variety of research questions. The questionnaire is economical in terms of both time and money as a large number of research respondents can be reached relatively quickly and easily. It is particularly useful for gathering information about people's attitudes and knowledge.

The interview

> Interviewing ... is not a research method but a family of research approaches that have only one thing in common – conversation between people in which one person has the role of the researcher. (Arksey and Knight 1999: 2)

Interviewing is one of the most personal of all research methods because the researcher and the research participant come into direct contact. Kvale (1996) refers to the interview as a 'professional conversation'. The interview can be used as the sole research method or as one of many methods in a multi-method approach. It can also be used as a means of gathering information prior to the main research project, for example to construct a questionnaire, or after other methods have been used to elaborate on issues in more depth.

Interviews can be highly structured, where they are little more than spoken questionnaires, or totally unstructured where they resemble an ordinary conversation. Most interviews fall somewhere between these two extremes and can be placed on the following continuum:

Structured.........Semi-structured.........Unstructured

The structured interview is also referred to as 'standardized', 'formal' and 'closed'; the unstructured interview as 'non-standardized', 'informal', 'open', and 'non-directive'. In this chapter the terms 'structured', 'semi-structured' and 'unstructured' will be used. Many of the issues pertaining to questionnaires in Chapter 8, for example the preparatory work involved and the wording of the questions, are very similar for the interview. You are advised to read Chapter 8 in conjunction with this chapter.

Stop and Think

Imagine that you are the parent of a 14-year-old girl who was supposed to get home by 11 pm but did not return until 3 am. In a few sentences, describe how you would take a structured, semi-structured and unstructured approach when talking to your daughter.

In a structured approach you would ask direct questions, for example 'Were you with Paul?', 'Did you go to a night club?', 'Why didn't you phone?' In a semi-structured approach your questions would be more open, for example 'Who were you with?', 'Where did you go?', 'What did you do?' In an unstructured approach you might say 'You were supposed to be in by eleven but now it's three. Tell me all about it.'

Structured interviews are associated with quantitative research, while semi-structured and unstructured interviews are associated with qualitative research.

The structured interview

In the structured interview the interviewer has control over the questions to be asked, the order in which they are asked, and the precise wording of the questions. The interviewer usually records the research participants' answers on an interview schedule which is a coding plan devised prior to the interview.

The interview schedule closely resembles a structured questionnaire, and may contain a variety of tick lists, scales and grids (see Chapter 8). The major difference is that research participants do not have to cope with the schedule themselves, so such factors as attractiveness of layout and ease of use are not so important. Great care must be taken over the wording of the questions to ensure that they do not unduly influence research participants' answers (see Chapter 8).

The semi-structured interview

With the semi-structured interview the interviewer knows what topics will be explored but is free to alter the wording and ordering of the questions with individual research participants. An interview schedule may be used but allowance will be made to record interesting and unique responses; often the interview schedule will merely consist of a list of questions. Although the subject matter of the interview is specified, research participants are given considerable freedom to express themselves as they wish. Researchers using this type of interview encourage research participants to expand on their answers by probing and prompting.

Numerous examples of semi-structured interviews can be found in the physiotherapy and occupational therapy literature. Teram et al (1999), for example, used semi-structured interviews with survivors of sexual abuse regarding the disclosure of their history to physiotherapists, and Murray (1998) used them to discover the effects on physiotherapy practice of therapists participating in a medical humanities group. Lister (1999) used them to discover the impact of being unable to drive, on people who had had a stroke, and Melton (1998) interviewed people with learning difficulties to evaluate some cookery sessions they had had with an occupational therapist. All of these studies had relatively few research participants but gathered rich and detailed data.

The unstructured interview

With this type of interview, no pre-planned set of questions are asked. Research participants are free to express themselves without being controlled or directed in any way. The interviewer can, however, raise queries and probe interesting points as they arise. The unstructured interview is commonly used in psychiatry and counselling but can be used for research, particularly at the early stages when the researcher is gathering ideas. Unstructured interviews, and to a lesser extent semi-structured interviews, can depend for their success on a reasonable level of articulacy on the part of research participants. Parr and Byng (1996), however, successfully interviewed people with severe aphasia, and Atkinson *et al* (1997) used interviews, together with other methods such as the use of photographs, with people with learning difficulties.

Stop and Think
Think of a time when you participated in an interview as a research participant or when you were interviewed by a professional such as a doctor. How structured was the interview? Did you feel constrained by the interview in any way? What do you consider to be the main advantages and disadvantages of the interviewing method you experienced?

Advantages and disadvantages of the structured interview

One of the advantages of the structured interview is that it tends to be quite brief and is therefore relatively inexpensive in terms of both time and money. It is also possible for the researcher to be assisted by other interviewers, after they have received appropriate training, as every research participant is asked exactly the same questions in the same order. Structured interviews are relatively easy to code and to replicate. As the wording and the order of the questions is the same in every interview, a high level of reliability is possible though validity may be compromised (Arksey and Knight, 1999).

Despite these advantages the structured interview has various limitations. As the questions are decided upon in advance, and researchers are required to restrict themselves to these questions, much potentially interesting material is lost. In addition, the constraints placed upon research participants may result in them feeling that the researcher is not interested in them as people, but merely as research objects. A further problem is that the same question wording may mean different things to different research participants, with some not understanding the question at all; despite this, researchers are not able to alter the question wording as they are with a less structured approach.

Advantages and disadvantages of the semi-structured and unstructured interview

Unstructured and semi-structured interviews are particularly useful when exploring relatively unknown material, when gathering in-depth information, and for learning about unique experiences, it is one of the method used, for example, by oral historians (see Chapter 16). The information obtained is very full and rich, unique responses are captured, and researchers are free to probe and follow up interesting points as they arise. In addition the content of each interview may be varied so that research participants can give the information they are best able to provide (Kvale, 1996).

The question wording and sequence may be changed to suit individual research participants; it is useful, for example, to be able to alter the wording when working with young children or people with a limited grasp of the researcher's language. In addition what is threatening to one research participant, and best left until the end of the interview when rapport has been established, may be fascinating to another who may feel frustrated if the topic is left until the end. Changing the wording and the sequence of questions may be thought to produce highly unreliable data, but as mentioned above, the same words can mean different things to different research participants, or may not be understood at all, so using the same words consistently does not necessarily ensure high reliability or validity.

In unstructured interviews the researcher will not have a list of questions to ask at all and in many semi-structured interviews the interview will be driven as much by the person being interviewed as by the interviewer. Rubin and Rubin (1995) liken the interview to a 'guided conversation' and believe that conversational skills and a relationship need to be built with research participants (or conversational partners as they call them) in order for a successful outcome. Reflection, on the part of the interviewer and the interviewee, is also important.

The researcher has little control over timing, so unstructured and semi-structured interviews tend to be expensive in terms of both time and money. It is also difficult to train other people to carry out the interviews as they need a very firm grasp of the subject matter in order to know which points to explore. Because of the freedom research participants are given to express themselves, topic areas tend to arise in a fairly haphazard fashion, yet imposing order on them may interfere with the free and natural flow of conversation which is one of the advantages of this approach. A further problem is that coding and analysing the data is difficult because it is so rich and diverse that it is not readily categorized. Interviewer bias, for example the way in which researchers phrase questions or their choice of issues to probe or ignore, is more likely to occur than in the structured interview and may influence the research participants' answers. Categorizing the responses is also subject to bias. Some researchers present a reflective account of the interviewing process in which they make public any ways in which they could have influenced the data (Seale and Barnard, 1998). Many qualitative researchers strongly advocate this reflective approach and advise researchers to keep a journal in which to record their thoughts and feelings concerning the research process and their role within it.

Although it can be useful to look at interview methods in terms of advantages and disadvantages, it is not entirely sensible to compare them in this way. Each method is chosen to reflect the researcher's research question or aim, and is built on a particular set of principles and philosophical assumptions pertaining to quantitative and qualitative research (see Chapters 1 and 15).

Interviewers can use a variety of approaches within the same interview. When interviewing research participants with cerebral palsy, for example, the therapist may require very structured, factual information regarding the treatment the research participants have received, but may want them to express themselves freely when talking about their own perceptions and feelings concerning the treatment.

> **Stop and Think**
> Devise a few questions to investigate a topic of your choice using a semi-structured interview. How open or closed are the questions you have written? Write a few words by each question which explains and justifies its inclusion.

Special types of interview

Specific types of interviews have been described which can be structured, semi-structured or unstructured.

The covert interview

In the covert interview the research participants do not know they are being interviewed; interviewers conceal their role while assuming another, for example the role of researcher may be concealed by the role of therapist. The advantage of covert interviews is that interviewers can obtain detailed and perhaps more honest information than they would in the conventional interview, though this will depend on the roles they are adopting. For example, a therapist may interview colleagues about their experiences during training by means of staff room conversation over a period of time.

The problem with covert interviewing is that researchers must interview in a way that is appropriate to their adopted role. As a result there are likely to be many questions which cannot be asked without arousing suspicion. This method also tends to be time-consuming because if researchers ask many questions on the same topic at any one time they will appear to be behaving strangely; in addition the deception involved in covert methods tends to place researchers under considerable stress.

Covert methods raise numerous ethical dilemmas and should

not be used without a great deal of thought and justification. The research participants may, for example, feel betrayed, and they will not have given their informed consent. Some people do believe that this type of interview is justified, however, if the investigation concerns discrimination or malpractice where the information required would not be forthcoming by the use of more conventional research methods. It is unlikely that undergraduate therapists would be given permission to conduct research of this type. (For details of ethical issues in research, see Chapter 3.)

The telephone interview

Interviewing over the telephone is a relatively inexpensive method most suitable if research participants are widely scattered geographically, or if a large number are being interviewed. Telephone interviews are usually, but not necessarily, highly structured and relatively impersonal (Arksey and Knight, 1999). People may be unwilling to discuss personal topics over the telephone and supplementary information, such as non-verbal communication and details of the research participant's surroundings, are not available. There may be sampling problems with telephone interviews as people without telephones cannot be included, and not everyone has their telephone number in the directory. It may also exclude some disabled people, for example deaf people and people with learning difficulties (Seale and Barnard, 1998). Telephone interviews can be recorded provided the permission of the research participant is obtained.

The group interview

Group interviews are invaluable if time and money are short as several research participants are interviewed at the same time and place. Sometimes group interviews are used to gather information prior to the main research project, for example to assist in constructing a questionnaire. Sometimes the group may be given an activity prior to the interview, for example watching some short extracts of video, to stimulate group discussion.

The major disadvantage of group interviews is that the dynamics of the group, for example the tendency people have to conform and the dominance of some people over others, may mean that the views expressed are not as diverse or valid as they might have been if research participants had been interviewed individually (Denscombe, 1998). The researcher may, however, be conducting group interviews as a way of studying group dynamics. Some people, for example children, may be less intimidated if interviewed in a group and ideas from one person may stimulate other people to contribute. This was the reason Jones and Tannock (2000) chose the group interview when investigating the understanding and experience of death and bereavement among primary school children. The data gathered from a group interview is likely to be different from that gathered from a number of people interviewed separately. This was found by Costley (2000) when interviewing groups of young people with moderate learning difficulties.

The focus group is a specialized group interview. Sim and Snell describe it as:

> ... a group interview centred on a specific topic ('focus') – and facilitated and co-ordinated by a moderator or facilitator – which seeks to generate primarily qualitative data, by capitalizing on the interaction that occurs within the group setting. (1986: 189)

There are frequently a series of groups each consisting of 8 to 12 people. The facilitator needs to be skilled at managing group dynamics though his or her input should be small.

Sim and Snell (1996) describe a series of focus groups comprised of patients attending a physiotherapy outpatient clinic. The aim was to help develop a patient-orientated outcome measurement tool. It was found that the patients had different conceptions about key concepts such as pain than the physiotherapists, and that they focused on the psychological benefits of physiotherapy treatment more than the physiotherapists did. Comments such as 'They keep you going' and 'She really gave me confidence' were common. (For a detailed account of focus groups, see Stewart and Shamdasani, 1990.)

> **Stop and Think**
> From your experience of research interviewing or clinical interviewing, make a list of the social, psychological and environmental factors that you consider necessary in order for the interview to be successful.

The social psychology of the interview

Interviewing, like any skill, must first be acquired and then improved upon with practice. Therapists carry out an enormous number of semi-structured clinical interviews in the course of their everyday work, so they should be at a considerable advantage compared with other new researchers. Practice may, however, be required. Carrying out a few trial research interviews which are recorded using a video camera or tape recorder, enables researchers to observe their own performances; this can help them improve their technique provided helpful and constructive feedback is given.

The interview is a social situation in which research participants are voluntarily giving their time. The researcher should arrange to conduct the interview at a time and in a place of the research participant's choosing. The researcher may wish to randomize the time and the place of the interviews, or alternatively keep the time and the place constant. For example, if some research participants were interviewed in the therapy department and others at home, their responses might be differentially affected by the environment. Similarly a therapist wishing to interview research participants about their symptoms may need to consider the timing of the interviews as some symptoms show a characteristic pattern throughout the day which could influence the research participants' replies; their symptoms may also be affected by a long journey. On the other hand, interviewing all the research participants last thing on a Friday afternoon, when they feel tired and are looking forward to the weekend, may introduce unnecessary distortions into the data.

Research participants are more likely to co-operate if they feel the research is worthwhile and if they know something about the person conducting it. Therapists should usually tell research participants of their profession, and therapy students should mention the institutions where they are studying. At all times the research participants need to be treated not merely as research participants but as human beings; the purpose of the interview should be explained, giving them sufficient time to understand, and they should be told how the results will be used and when and where they will be available for inspection. The researcher should also ask the research participant's permission to use the tape recorder and should explain how the information will be safeguarded. Neglecting these issues amounts to unethical practice. Many researchers like to give research participants a copy of their interview transcript for comment, or to produce an interim report for discussion. This involves research participants more actively, and is a means of checking the validity of the data.

Research participants need to be assured that their responses will remain confidential and anonymous. If they are not convinced of this it is unlikely that they will be entirely truthful or open. Alternatively, the researcher may ask the research participants if they require the data from their interview to remain confidential and anonymous. If research participants are well-known or unusual people, it can be difficult ensuring that they are not identifiable in research reports.

Non-verbal communication

In most types of interview therapists will come face to face with research participants. The research participants' non-verbal communication can be a useful additional source of knowledge, but it can distort verbal information as well as enhance it. Lack of facial expression or a monotonous voice, for instance, may give therapists the impression that research participants are uninterested or unintelligent, which in turn may affect their own behaviour, possibly distorting the data. Silences tend to be embarrassing and often seem much longer than they really are. Researchers need to remember that the subject matter of the interview, though familiar to them, may be new to research participants who may need time to think. It is advisable for researchers to record their impressions of non-verbal information and aspects of the environment as soon as the interview is complete.

Researchers may influence what research participants say and how they behave, not only by their verbal input, but by their non-verbal communication. A bored expression, or a hint of exasperation in the voice, for example, will be readily detected by research participants, possibly leading to an alteration in their behaviour. Problems such as these can be reduced with training, but there are various characteristics known to affect research participants' responses which are difficult or impossible to change, such as gender, age, accent, status and personality (May, 1997).

Uniforms are another source of non-verbal communication; they give information regarding occupation and status and may also engender feelings of respect, fear, diffidence or trust. They also tend to create a psychological distance between the researcher and the research participant. Therapists will need to consider the benefits and drawbacks of wearing a uniform to interview; this will, in part, depend on the research participants and the purpose of the interview.

The physical environment

The interview should ideally take place in an environment where privacy is assured and where neither the research participant nor the researcher will be distracted. An office with a telephone, or a room where people are free to come and go is best avoided.

The physical arrangement of the furniture, and the distance between the researcher and research participant are also important. If, for example, the researcher sits some distance from the research participant and interposes a desk between them the atmosphere will tend to be rather formal, especially if they are sitting directly facing each other. A less formal arrangement can be achieved by removing the table and sitting closer, though not too close, to the research participant, and at right angles rather than face to face. The interview is likely to be an unusual interruption of everyday routine for research participants and they may not, therefore, be displaying their usual behaviour.

The social and psychological environment

When interviewing it is essential that the researcher appears interested in the topic; this may be easy for the first five or six interviews, but can become difficult by the nineteenth or twentieth even though the researcher may be very committed to the topic under investigation. The interviewer needs to be sensitive and provide an empathic and non-judgemental atmosphere. Therapists who have developed counselling skills and experience may be at a considerable advantage as many interviewing techniques are similar to those required of the counsellor. The interview should not be allowed to drag, but the research participants need to be given sufficient time to think about the questions before answering. An effort must be made not to influence research participants' answers by either verbal or non-verbal behaviour.

Researchers must do everything they can to minimize the 'social desirability' effect. This refers to the tendency people have to present themselves in as favourable a light as possible. Research participants may feel that various aspects of their lives will discredit them in the eyes of the researcher, for example unemployment and personal habits such as smoking. If researchers hold strong views on some issue, they need to reflect on the part they play in the construction of the research process rather than pretending that they are neutral.

The social desirability effect has been shown to threaten the validity of research, but researchers can minimize it by paying close attention to the wording of questions and by creating a friendly and empathic environment. The relationship with research participants can, however, be problematic and skill is needed to strike the right balance.

Ending interviews can also be difficult especially if there has been a series with the same research participants over a period of time, and if the research participants found them rewarding. With isolated groups, such as some people with learning difficulties, this can give rise to significant ethical dilemmas (Atkinson, 1993).

Researchers should endeavour to avoid the 'halo effect'. This effect occurs when researchers allow one piece of information about the research participant, for example something which is said, or the environment in which the interview takes place, such as an unkempt home, to colour everything else about the research participant. There is a tendency to make global inferences about people on the basis of very little information and to underestimate just how much people's behaviour is affected by the situation and environment they are in.

The pilot study

Before the interviews are undertaken it is important to run two or three trial interviews to eliminate any problems that may have been overlooked. Pilot interviews may also suggest additional questions and topics that need to be explored. If researchers have taken care in designing the interview schedule, problems should not be difficult to resolve.

Organizing the interviews

Stop and Think
Imagine that you have to organize ten interviews during one week when you are working. What factors will you take into account to ensure that the operation runs smoothly?

Carrying out a number of interviews, especially when they are geographically spread, requires meticulous organization. If time or money are short it is tempting to squeeze as many interviews as possible into a day, or to travel about hoping and praying that traffic will not be heavy or that public transport will not let you down. Something is bound to go wrong, however, and it is important that you anticipate this rather than losing research participants unnecessarily because you were late, or because you did not write or telephone to confirm the time and place of the interview. Make sure that your tape recorder is in good order and that you have some spare batteries and tapes. An extension lead can also be invaluable.

Analysing the data

Quantitative data

Quantitative data is analysed by means of descriptive and inferential statistics (see Chapter 15).

Qualitative data

If the interviews were tape-recorded the researcher should transcribe them from the tape into a verbatim script. This process is very time-consuming. Transcribing is something a competent typist can cope with although going through the data in detail can be beneficial to the researcher in beginning to make sense of it (May, 1997). Qualitative interview data is analysed by means of content analysis and other qualitative approaches which are discussed in Chapter 15.

Conclusion

When compared with other methods the interview has a number of very important advantages; indeed it is often the only suitable research method available. It is more personal and enjoyable than most methods and the response rate is higher than that of the questionnaire (Domholdt, 2000). This is probably because talking is less of an effort than writing and most people enjoy expressing their views to an interested person.

The structured interview can be useful when the researcher wants to meet the research participants or when they are unlikely to complete a questionnaire. Semi-structured and unstructured interviews are ideal for gathering detailed, rich information about research participants' experiences, feelings and attitudes. They enable people to put forward their views without being constrained by the perspectives and agenda of the researcher. Self-reflection on the part of the researcher is, however, necessary in understanding and revealing their role in creating the knowledge produced.

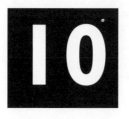

The Delphi technique

The Delphi technique is a research method used to gather and analyse the opinions of a group of people who are frequently experts in a particular field. This is achieved by sending sequential questionnaires to each research participant (Domholdt, 2000). The Delphi technique is often used as a means of forecasting future events to circumvent problems. Stewart and Shamdasani (1990) explain that the name of this technique derives from the Oracles of Delphi in ancient Greek literature who, it is claimed, could see into the future. The strength of the Delphi technique lies in its ability to portray consensus or, conversely, to expose differing points of view.

The Delphi technique will be briefly explained by describing a study by Green (1996). The topic under investigation was the role of the occupational therapist in enabling people to make vocational choices following illness and injury. The research participants in the study were service users, employment service workers, GPs, hospital consultants and people working in voluntary associations and training agencies. The 35 research participants were asked to fill in three sequential questionnaires.

The first questionnaire

The first questionnaire was open-ended. The research participants were simply asked to list up to five problems that people had when returning to work after illness or injury. The data was then collected and collated by the researchers; 37 problems were identified.

The second questionnaire

A second questionnaire was then devised listing all the problems which had been identified in the first questionnaire. It was sent to the same research participants who were asked to rank the five items that they considered to be most important. The five items that were rated, overall, as most important were financial problems, loss of confidence, coping with disability, employers' attitudes, and training.

The third questionnaire

In the third and final questionnaire the research participants were asked for their open-ended comments on the five items identified in the second round. Their comments were then analysed by the researchers.

Using the Delphi technique in therapy research

The Delphi technique could be used to answer a variety of questions of interest and concern to therapists. In every case the overall format would be similar to that of Green's investigation, but the details of each study would be unique. There may, for example, be four rather than three rounds of questionnaires and the research participants may be asked to consider particular problems in different ways.

A physiotherapy tutor, for example, could use the Delphi technique to discover how clinical educators perceive the effectiveness of massage as a therapeutic treatment, and whether it should still be taught to physiotherapy students. Using this as an example, in the first questionnaire the research participants may be asked to list the benefits and drawbacks of massage as they perceive them. Some may, for example, mention an enhancement of the placebo effect, the benefits of physical contact, and the physiological effects of massage, while others may believe that massage is too time-consuming and that it encourages passivity on the part of patients. In the second questionnaire these views could be listed and the research participants asked to indicate those that they consider to be important.

In the third and final questionnaire, all the items from the second questionnaire, which were ticked by at least two thirds of the research participants, could be listed. At this point the researcher might decide to combine some of the items if they are perceived to be very similar. For example an item 'It helps patients to relax' could be combined with 'It reduces tension', and an item 'It takes too long' could be combined with 'It is not cost effective'. There is a danger when combining items that meanings are distorted, and that valuable information may be lost and researcher bias introduced. One way of reducing this problem is to involve others, perhaps the research participants themselves, in the analysis of the data.

In the third questionnaire the research participants could be asked for their opinions on each item and whether, on balance, they believe that massage should be retained in physiotherapy education.

Stop and Think
Think of a research question of interest to you where the Delphi technique could be applied. Briefly describe the study noting down what the research participants would be asked to do at each stage.

Cross (1999) reports on the first two rounds of a Delphi study which set out to discover the differing views of lecturers and clinical teachers on the attributes of a 'good' and a 'bad' clinical physiotherapy student. 113 university-based physiotherapy academics and 108 senior physiotherapy practitioners took part in the study. The purpose of the study was to help develop guidelines for assessing students in their clinical practice.

In the first round the research participants were asked to

provide between ten and twenty adjectives or adjectival phrases to describe 'good' and 'bad' clinical physiotherapy students. Many of the adjectives overlapped and were combined into single categories by the researcher. A total of 24 categories describing a 'good' clinical physiotherapy student, and 25 categories describing a 'bad' clinical physiotherapy student remained following this analysis.

In the second round of the study the research participants were provided with these two lists of categories and were asked to rank their 'top ten' for each list. There was a large degree of agreement between the two groups of research participants which was highly statistically significant. Differences were, however, found between them. The academics, for example, included 'critical thinking' and 'independent learner' more often than the clinicians who showed a greater preference for 'good record keeping' and 'common sense'.

Advantages and disadvantages of the Delphi technique

Stop and Think
Look back at the Delphi study you devised in activity 1. What do you think are the particular advantages and disadvantages of using this method to answer your research question?

The value of the Delphi technique is that all the research participants are provided with feedback concerning the views of others, which gives them the opportunity to take into account aspects of the problem which they may not have considered. It might be thought that this could be achieved just as effectively through group discussion, but a major advantage of the Delphi technique is that each participant has an equal voice. As Babbie explains:

The key is that participants can contribute equally – they don't know which comment is from the boss and which is from the mail clerk – and since no one knows what they said initially, they can change their minds without losing face. (1992: 486)

The Delphi technique is a useful means of obtaining a consensus viewpoint rather than the researcher collating all the shared themes. The strategy can also stimulate reflective thought which the research participants may not be able to achieve if given a single questionnaire. These processes are well illustrated in a four round Delphi study by Sumsion (1999) which sought to determine a definition of client-centred practice among British occupational therapists.

The Delphi technique can provide a way of engaging a wide range of opinion in an efficient and cost-effective manner. Hitch and Murgatroyd state:

It combines the virtue of the mail survey (lack of interviewer contamination, time to sit down and ponder, no travelling costs) with those of a meeting (where the whole is greater than the parts). The Delphi technique is relatively inexpensive in terms of both time and money; it is far easier to send out questionnaires than to arrange for a large number of people to meet together several times, it can also involve more people than would be feasible in a face-to-face meeting. (1983: 422)

When people discuss issues in a group, many psychological forces, known as group dynamics, operate to shape their responses. People have a tendency to conform to the majority view, with some being more confident and dominant than others. Groups also tend to take riskier decisions than individuals, possibly because of a diffusion of responsibility. The larger the group the less likely are some members to contribute, while others are reluctant to state a view before they have all the facts before them. In addition homogeneous groups may be cohesive but have a restricted range of ideas, whereas heterogeneous groups may have many more ideas but be antagonistic (Brown, 1988).

These problems are, to some extent, avoided if the Delphi technique is used (Domholdt, 2000). The research participants do not meet and all remain anonymous, but they have the benefit of receiving information from each other to help them develop their own views and reach decisions. Beretta (1996) contends, however, that lack of discussion can be regarded as a disadvantage of the Delphi technique.

The Delphi technique is also effective in terms of time and cost as a large number of people can contribute relatively cheaply and easily. Beretta states that:

> The Delphi technique is a research method which combines qualities of the postal questionnaire in covering a potentially wide population, and the committee meeting in bringing together expert opinion. (1996: 87)

One criticism levelled against the Delphi technique is its use of 'experts' as research participants. Deciding who the real experts are is never straightforward; people perceived as experts are frequently specialists whose views are sometimes blinkered and who may form a tight-knit, homogeneous group. Linstone and Turoff (1975) point out that a single person may have greater insight than all the experts put together, a fact which is amply demonstrated in the history of science. The criticism is not too problematic, however, because non-experts can be used as research participants without affecting the efficiency or the structure of the technique. Service users were, for example, included in the study by Green (1996).

In devising subsequent rounds of the questionnaire the researcher may disregard minority views and opinions. In the study by Green (1996) on the employment problems of people who had been ill or injured, for example, the five items that were rated collectively as most important by the research participants were used in the second round of questionnaires. At this point, therefore, minority views may have been disregarded even though they may have had value, especially in complex areas of practice. People whose views are not represented in early rounds may feet alienated and drop out of the study.

The psychological processes which operate when people meet in a group are not altogether lacking when people are presented with questionnaires, as they are with the Delphi technique. There may, for example, still be a tendency to conform

(Seale and Barnard, 1998) and the 'social desirability effect' whereby people strive to be seen in a favourable light by others, may still operate. In addition the research participants' views may be affected by knowing who the other research participants are, even if they are not known by name. Indeed in a fairly tight-knit group, for example physiotherapy or occupational therapy lecturers, it is likely that people will know each other and may discuss the questionnaires (Beretta, 1996). The decisions of the research participants will also be specific to the particular time and culture in which they live; they may, for example, be influenced by the media or by current professional debates. A further problem which is common to all measures of attitude and opinion, is that what people say they do may not tally with what they actually do.

It is necessary, if the Delphi technique is to work well, that the research participants are sufficiently motivated to fill in several questionnaires; it is perhaps inevitable that some research participants will be lost. Research participants also need a good level of written expression which may eliminate some people from the research, although in some studies verbal expression using a cassette recorder has been used as an alternative to a written account (Beretta, 1996).

Another problem is preserving the momentum of the study; delays need to be kept to a minimum but this is not always easy, especially when a large number of research participants are involved. Beretta (1996) estimates that 45 days are required for each round of questionnaires.

Conclusion

The Delphi technique is not as well known as some research methods but it is well worth considering as a means of investigating certain research questions that therapists may confront. It is a means of gathering together a large range of opinions relatively quickly and easily and of giving research participants the benefit of each others' ideas and opinions while minimizing the social and psychological effect of meeting face to face.

Experimental and quasi-experimental research

The experimental method is highly prized, particularly by physical and medical scientists. This is because, in contrast with surveys, observations and interview methods, the experiment can (at least potentially) establish cause and effect. Whilst the non-experimental methods may *suggest* causal influences, only a well-designed experimental study can provide really strong *evidence* about such influences. Experimental research tests hypotheses. Imagine that therapists decide to offer a given pain management treatment within a group setting rather than to individual patients. On the basis of their clinical experiences, they hypothesize that the 'group' treatment A reduces long-term disability more effectively than the 'individual' treatment B. This is known as the experimental hypothesis (or 'alternate' hypothesis). The measured outcomes of the treatments also test the 'null' hypothesis which states that there is no difference in responses to experimental and the control conditions (apart from small variation linked to chance factors). Further discussion of hypothesis-testing is provided in Chapter 4 and Chapter 12. Experimental methods can provide sound evidence about the relative effectiveness of different interventions.

An experiment examines the effects of applying a well specified intervention or influence of some sort to a random set of participants.

Independent variable   ➔   Dependent variable
(influencing variable)   (outcome variable)

The influencing variable is termed the 'independent variable', or IV. The participants' measured response (physical, behavioural or otherwise) is termed the 'dependent variable', or DV (as the magnitude of the response is considered to 'depend' on the independent variable). A useful mnemonic for remembering the difference between IV and DV is that 'independent variable' begins with the same letters as influence or intervention.

As discussed in Chapter 1, a variable represents a single dimension. An important skill in experimental research is identifying the many variables that operate in a given situation. When assessing outcomes of the experiment, attention needs to be given to establishing reliable, valid measures of each experimental variable. As there may be many possible effects of an experimental manipulation, it will be necessary for the experimenter to determine firstly whether to measure one or more variables, and then to decide which measures to select. Variables generally require operational definitions, as discussed in Chapter 1. As well as making sense conceptually, the IV and DV have to be measurable. For example, studies of the effectiveness of pain treatments require a suitable self-report measure. A validated measure such as the McGill pain inventory may be appropriate. A measure of functional status, such as the Barthel scale may be selected to document change in independent activities. Some experimenters measure several DVs (outcomes), but data analysis can become very challenging if too many are selected. It is usually good practice to select the measures that have been shown to be sensitive and appropriate in previously published relevant research.

Although it is usual for all variables to be measured quantitatively, the experimental method does not *require* quantification. It may be possible for example to assess participants' responses to different experimental conditions through qualitative interviews. For example, Biggerstaff *et al* (2000) carried out an experimental comparison of women's experiences of different forms of post-natal care, in part through qualitative interview data. A mixed-method approach to data collection may have particular relevance to establishing clinical effectiveness. Both objective as well as subjective evaluation can test the usefulness of a therapeutic approach.

Stop and Think

Identify the IV and DV in the studies outlined below:

1. The anxiety levels of two randomly selected groups of patients with hip replacements were compared one day after their operations. Pre-operatively, the 'experimental' group had received the usual treatment and also some additional information about coping with pain. The control group had received the usual treatment without the educational session:

   IV=   DV=

2. Patients with multiple sclerosis were either treated as out-patients or as in-patients on an otherwise identical rehabilitation programme. Measures of independence in Activities of Daily Living (ADL) and depression were taken immediately after the treatment programme and again six months later.

   IV=   DVI=   DV2=

In (1) above, the IV is presence/absence of the educational session, and the DV is anxiety.

In (2) above, the IV is in-patient/out-patient treatment. There are two DVs – independence in ADL and depression, measured at two time intervals (four measures altogether).

Experimental design: dealing with confounding variables

Experiments investigate the effect of one variable (IV) on another (the DV). To do this convincingly, other potentially influential variables have to be held constant (controlled).

Stop and Think

Therapists in a multi-disciplinary team treating out-patients with low back pain had a hunch that patients who received both educational and exercise aspects of treatment in groups were making more progress than those treated on a one-to-one basis. For example, compared with individually treated patients, those treated in a group had reported less pain, and showed greater mobility at the end of the programme. Without conducting a controlled trial, the therapists concluded that the social element of the treatment was responsible for the enhanced outcome.

This is a risky conclusion because many other variables could be responsible for the outcomes noted. Can you identify at least two variables (apart from social contact) that could be responsible for the different measured outcomes of patients treated in groups or individually?

Many variables in this hypothetical scenario could account for different patient outcomes:

- Diagnosis/severity: if the patients initially assessed as having less severe pain were allocated to group treatment (rather than individually tailored treatment) they may 'appear' to respond better to the therapeutic programme.
- Age: if the 'group' patients were younger than the patients treated individually, they may return to health and strength more quickly (regardless of the intervention context).
- Time in treatment: if the treatment for group patients was offered over more weeks, then the passage of time itself might be responsible for improved progress.
- Therapist: if group treatment was carried out by Therapist A and individual treatment by Therapist B, then factors such as therapist experience and/or enthusiasm might account for different responses in the two patient groups.
- Volunteering/self-selection: if patients personally decided upon their preferred approach to treatment, then those opting for group treatment may be rather different in per-

sonality, coping styles and so on. These factors rather than treatment modality itself, could account for different outcomes.

This list of *confounding variables* which could account for observed outcomes is not exhaustive. However, it demonstrates the complexity of measuring the effect of a single IV upon behaviour or physical functioning.

Stop and Think
If you were experimentally to compare the effectiveness of group versus individual treatment (IV) for low back pain (DV), what variables would you want to keep constant (or similar) in the two groups?

You would need to control for the variables relating to diagnosis/severity. Any variable apart from the IV that is thought to affect the DV in question should be kept constant as far as possible during the experiment. For example, the same therapists should preferably be involved in treating each set of patients.

So what is a *control group*? A control group experiences all variables apart from the IV under investigation. However, in a clinical setting, it is generally unethical to withhold treatment so the control group cannot usually consist of patients receiving 'nothing'. In some studies, the control group is selected from patients on the existing waiting list for treatment. In other studies, the control group is made up of patients receiving the usual or standard treatment, and the experimental group receives the new treatment whose additional efficacy is being evaluated. In the above example, the control patients may be treated 'normally', i.e. individually. However, if following a genuine experimental design, the therapist-researcher would ensure that control and experimental (group) patients share similar diagnoses, initial severity of reported pain, the same therapist, continue for the same number of sessions and weeks, and so on. If the patients treated in groups continued to show more progress than those receiving individual treatment, the evidence for the effectiveness of a group approach would be much stronger.

You may already have questioned whether therapists in the clinical setting can really arrange control groups, and the ethics of doing so. In realistic settings (in contrast to artificial laboratory environments) it is also extremely difficult to control or eliminate all extraneous variables. For these reasons, the experimental approach is usually adapted as a *randomized controlled trial* (RCT) for evaluating treatment effectiveness. Patients are randomly allocated into alternative treatments, and their responses are assessed and compared with baseline measures. The alternative treatments may comprise a number of 'independent variables', so less precise determination of cause and effect is generally possible than in a 'true' experiment. Nevertheless the RCT design is accepted as providing a robust approach to determining treatment effectiveness, and many literature reviews now selectively focus on RCT outcomes. Another practical approach to treatment evaluation is provided by quasi-experimental designs, and these will be considered later.

Pre-testing and post-testing

To examine change, the DV may be measured before and after the participants engage in the experimental or control conditions. This is known as pre- and post-testing. In other designs, sometimes participants are only compared on measures taken during or after the experiment – known as post-testing only. Pre- and post-testing allows tracking of individual change, whereas post-testing only permits comparison between the groups in each condition. If there is more change in the experimental group than the control group, and if that change is found to be statistically significant, then it is concluded that the independent variable brought about the change.

Double-blind testing

It is usual to keep patients unaware of the hypothesis being tested. In a *double-blind* experimental design, even the researchers who administer the treatments and the researchers who analyse the data do not know which participant has received the experimental treatment and which has received the control treatment. This approach is very common in drug versus placebo trials. The precaution helps to avoid bias, as researchers (and indeed participants) can behave in subtly different ways if aware of the hypothesis being tested and the condition in which a patient is participating.

Random allocation of participants

Genuine experiments can only establish cause and effect when all confounding variables have been excluded. One important way of doing this is through random selection of participants. Firstly, the sample of participants should be taken at random from the population of interest to the study. Secondly, the sample should be randomly allocated to the different experimental and control conditions.

Random allocation helps to ensure that there is an equivalent mixture of abilities, needs, strengths, coping styles and so on in each group being compared. Non-random methods such as patients volunteering to enter one condition or another, or being allocated by therapists according to assessed need, will bias the data as the two groups being compared are already clearly different at the outset, even before experiencing the IV. (See Chapter 7 on sampling for further information.)

Experimental design: comparing participants

There are three main design options for allocating participants to conditions:

'Same subjects' – 'repeated measures – 'within groups' – related design: These terms are used interchangeably. In this design, participants experience both (or all) conditions. They act as their own controls, by participating in the control condition as well as the experimental condition. If there are two different experimental conditions, the sample participates in both. In some clinical evaluations, the repeated measure design may be achieved by documenting any change in patients' status whilst on a placebo treatment (the control condition), and then comparing progress during the active treatment (the experimental condition). To keep control over confounding variables in this design, half of the subjects need to experience condition A before B and half should experience B before A – a counterbalanced or 'crossover' design.

Half of the sample: Condition A   →   Condition B
Half of the sample: Condition B   →   Condition A

In this way, the experimenter acquires some control over 'order effects'. Order effects occur because patients take their experiences (including the skills and knowledge that they learn) from the first condition to the second.

Stop and Think
Imagine that the relative efficacy of relaxation versus exercise was compared for people with persistent low back pain. The design was poor because *all* patients started with four weekly sessions of exercise and ended with a similar number of relaxation sessions. If participants report more marked reductions in pain during the first treatment phase, the therapist should *not* conclude that exercise was the more efficacious treatment. Why not? Think of at least two 'order' effects that may make the first phase of treatment more effective, regardless of treatment modality.

There are many reasons why patients respond quickly to the initial therapeutic input – they may feel relieved to receive help and validation of their pain, they may receive social support from therapists and other patients, they may learn from the educational material handed out to all new patients. All of these experiences may provide a sense of hope that pain can be coped with and made more tolerable. None of these effects would be specific to the exercise classes. A more robust experimental design would involve half of the patients undergoing treatment in the reverse order: relaxation for 4 weeks then exercise. If the patients continued to show more gains during exercise (whatever its position in the treatment programme) there would be more grounds for concluding that this intervention is particularly effective.

Some related designs compare the changes shown by participants whilst on a waiting list with their progress during treatment. However, it is clearly impossible to achieve a counterbalanced design as patients cannot sensibly undergo treatment *followed by* a waiting list control condition. A quasi-experimental design may be required to resolve this problem, and some further design strategies will be considered later. Nevertheless, there are some published studies which report patients following a period of active treatment with 'no' treatment. For example, Taylor (1999) looked at the response of patients with mild-to-moderate chronic heart failure to a mild exercise programme. Those who underwent 8 weeks of exercise followed by 8 weeks of no-exercise showed a rapid loss of their gains in physical fitness in the control half of the programme. Whilst the experimental design provides convincing evidence of the physiological and psychological benefits of exercise for these patients, it also raises ethical issues. An intervention that deliberately deters patients from exercise resulting in loss of fitness may be considered to pose risk of harm.

The repeated measures design has many advantages. Because the performance of each individual can be compared in each condition, the design is sensitive to individual changes. Each individual essentially acts as his or her own control so the design does not require careful selection of 'similar' individuals in each group. Because individual change is documented, sample sizes generally can be smaller than with the unrelated design described below. However, sometimes individuals cannot participate in two conditions, because their response to the second condition is irrevocably modified by the effects of the first condition.

Matched subjects/matched pairs design: This is a particular form of repeated measures design, in which there are two groups of participants. Each participant is matched on key variables with a participant in the other condition. For example, pairs may be matched on age, sex, and disability/pain measures. The experimenter will examine whether participants in one condition make more progress than their matched counterparts in the other condition. Whilst the design has the advantages noted above, it is not particularly popular for two main reasons. Firstly, it can take time to match participants on the necessary variables. In clinical settings in particular, there is pressure to treat patients and it may not be ethical to leave patients to languish on a waiting list whilst a 'matched' partner is found. Secondly, there may be many other relevant variables other than those being matched. For example, two patients may be 40 years old, female, married and with similar reported levels of pain associated with rheumatoid arthritis. They are randomly allocated to different treatments. Despite this 'matching', the women may be very different in coping styles, social support, paid occupations and so on. These uncontrolled factors could have a strong (but unmeasured) influence on their response to treatment.

Different subjects – independent measures – unrelated – between groups design: These alternative terms describe possibly the most straightforward experimental design, involving different groups of participants in each condition. Their responses (functional, psychological and so on) are compared statistically to see whether the groups respond differently in each condition. In this design, there is no need for counterbalancing of order, as patients only experience one condition.

Group A   Pre-test   →   Treatment A   →   Post-test
Group B   Pre-test   →   Treatment B/Control   →   Post-test

For example, Munin *et al* (1998) randomly assigned eligible patients having total hip or knee replacements to one of two treatment programmes. One group began in-patient rehabilitation on day 3 following their operation, and the other group began their rehabilitation on day 7. Checks were made that baseline measures of function and health prior to surgery were similar in the two groups. This design enabled the researchers to determine that earlier rehabilitation conferred short-term (but not longer-term) advantages for patients' recovery.

The independent groups design has some advantages. There is no need for matching participants, or counterbalancing of conditions. However, the design depends on random allocation of participants to each condition. If the two groups are dissimilar at the start of the experiment, post-test results will reflect these initial differences, as well as the effects of the experimental/control conditions. In clinical studies, there are ethical problems in leaving some patients on a waiting list or placebo condition, simply for comparison purposes. A quasi-experimental design may be a preferred alternative.

Quasi-experimental designs

Although it is important for therapists to understand the principles of experimental design, it is relatively unusual for genuine experiments to be carried out in the clinical setting. This is because it may be impossible (practically and ethically) for patients:

● To be randomly allocated to treatment conditions.
● To be given no treatment or a placebo in a control condition.

A set of designs, known as quasi-experimental, provide strong alternatives (Johnston, Ottenbacher & Reichardt, 1995). Essentially these designs provide a mid-way stage between non-experimental (non-interventionist) and fully experimental research. There are many such designs and only one of the most straightforward is considered here.

Time-series designs follow patients up over time. *Repeated base-line measures* (of the selected outcome variable) are taken *prior* to treatment, often over several weeks, so that any spontaneous changes (associated with biological healing or deterioration, for example) can be determined. Then the treatment is introduced, and further repeated assessments of the DV are carried out. Any change in the DV which then follows the introduction of treatment, provides evidence for its effectiveness. Whilst this design can provide evidence that change occurs following the start of treatment, it remains possible that such change is occurring because of factors outside of treatment. For example, patients may coincidentally attempt a new strategy of coping with their condition through receiving new information via the mass media or from a patient support organization. This 'outside' influence could potentially be responsible for the measured change. As in 'true' experiments, identification of possible 'outside' influences can be achieved through the addition of a control group. If a similar set of assessments is carried out over time with a similar (control) group of patients who do not receive the 'active' treatment, any differences in the outcomes at the end of the entire evaluation period provide support for the effectiveness of treatment.

Some further potential problems in time-series designs can be encountered. Repeated testing can lead to practice or fatigue/boredom effects among participants. Such 'testing effects' may distort the data gathered, leading to over- or underestimates of the effects of treatment. Also, the time series design is longitudinal in nature. As with all longitudinal studies, there is a considerable risk of participants dropping out of the study as time progresses. The control group is particularly likely to become less representative of patients with the given condition. For example, if the more affluent patients on a lengthy waiting list become disillusioned and opt out, seeking private treatment, the remaining patients will represent a narrower income band (and range of social class) than the original sample. Conversely, if only the most motivated remain in the treatment condition, the treatment's real effectiveness may be overestimated.

Despite these problems, the multiple-group time-series design can provide reasonably robust evidence about the effectiveness of an intervention. However, caution should be exercised in generalizing the outcomes to other populations.

Further examples of naturalistic (rather than true) experiments occur when the researcher selects groups already different on a key variable, rather than deliberately subjecting them to an experimentally manipulated IV. A study that compared the responses of male and female patients (or smokers and non-smokers) to a relaxation programme would have a naturalistic experimental design. Neither gender nor smoking status are directly manipulated, but these variables can be regarded as an independent variable.

Single case designs

Apart from economy of scale, there are two particular advantages of researching the effects of treatment on single patients, rather than groups. Therapists are already familiar with assessing the individual's needs and priorities, formulating an appropriate intervention, and evaluating change, as part of their role. Also, patients with similar diagnoses (especially in the field of head injury and neurological conditions) may vary considerably in their intact skills and impairments. Grouping these patients and averaging their responses can mask these important individual differences.

Some single case designs resemble the time series quasi-experimental design, with baseline measures being taken over time prior to treatment, and then continued during and after treatment. This is sometimes known as the AB design. If changes occur in the 'B' phase, this provides some evidence of effectiveness. However, the baseline data (A) need to be stable in order to provide comparison. Without stability, no change can convincingly be demonstrated. The design lacks power because improvement in the treatment (B) phase cannot be readily distinguished from maturation/time influences.

Stronger designs are generally referred to as the ABA and ABAB designs. The placebo/no treatment condition (A) is alternated with the active treatment B, and checks are made whether the measured outcomes vary in line with the introduction and withdrawal of active treatment. For example, Crocker, MacKay-Lyons and McDonnell (1997) planned an intervention for a child more affected by cerebral palsy (CP) on one side of her body. They examined whether immobilizing the better functioning hand through splinting would lead to the child making more use of her less functional hand. They adopted an ABA design, with a 2-weeks pre-splinting (control) phase to obtain baseline measures, three weeks of splinting the hand less affected by CP (experimental phase) and then two weeks post-splinting (control phase again). The post-splinting measures showed that the child had learned to make greater use of the hand more affected by CP. Improvements continued to occur over the next four months (follow-up phase).

A major advantage of single case experiments is that they integrate research with clinical practice, thereby encouraging therapists to undertake research. Single case studies can be applied flexibly, give therapists and patients immediate feedback of the results of interventions, and the findings can be put into practice immediately. In addition, single case studies may be the only feasible way of applying experimental research to patients and clients with rare diseases or unusual problems. Even with some common conditions (such as stroke), patients are notoriously heterogeneous, throwing doubt on the validity of many large group experiments. Single case experimental studies are also less time-consuming and expensive than large scale studies.

The single case design has some disadvantages. Cause and effect can only be demonstrated convincingly if performance decreases during the second control (A) phase of the ABA design. This does not necessarily occur, especially if the patient has learned useful skills during the B phase which can be used in subsequent phases. Also, such experimental findings should not be generalized beyond the individual. The problem of lack of generalization may be overcome by repeating single case studies on many individuals, that is to carry out a case series. Single case experimentation can be less objective if the therapist is involved in both the intervention and the outcome evaluation. This problem can be overcome to some degree, however, by involving someone else in the evaluation of the treatment, at least some of the time.

You may have queried the ethics of the single case study described above. Patients should always be told that they are taking part in an experiment, but as the single case study is so bound up with clinical practice, such considerations may sometimes be overlooked or wrongly considered unnecessary. Similarly the studies may be carried out with no consultation with ethics committees on the grounds that such tests are merely an aspect of the patient's treatment. Yet ABA designs often raise ethical concerns because they involve the withholding of treatment in the A phases. Additional discussion of ethical issues is given in Chapter 3.

Conclusion

Classic experimental research is a very powerful means of establishing causal relationships. However, 'pure' experiments can be difficult to design and carry out, particularly in clinical settings. Quasi-experimental designs are often more practicable. The single case study, in particular, is believed by many therapists and researchers to offer an effective approach to experimental research in clinical settings. Ethical issues need careful consideration in all treatment evaluations, especially those which involve withholding treatment in control conditions.

Despite the strength of the method, care must be taken when inferring cause and effect. Whilst the experiment can demonstrate differences in the performance of experimental and control groups, the precise reasons for such differences are not always clear. A given 'independent variable' may be experienced in many different ways by participants, and this is rarely checked. Earlier in the chapter a hypothetical scenario was presented in which a 'group' intervention was more effective than an 'individual' programme. Additional qualitative enquiry might reveal that the group programme was beneficial for some participants because they viewed it as offering social support, whereas for others it stimulated healthy competition. Careful examination of all data might even reveal a subgroup of patients performing *less* well in the group setting because they felt demeaned or embarrassed. Qualitative methods can enable the researcher to make further enquiry into patient's experiences, and their subjective views of why and how they are responding to treatment. These are considered further in other chapters.

Observation

Observation is a research method where the researcher studies behaviour mainly by watching and listening, either from the outside or by participating in the activities under investigation. It is suitable for investigating many types of behaviour, as well as the environment in which the behaviour takes place. Observation is part of everyday life and is integral to social interaction. When observation is used as a research method, however, it requires a more systematic, reflective approach.

Observation can be used as the main research tool, as one method among others in a multi-method approach, or as a means of gathering general data prior to the main research project. Most research methods contain some observation (Banister *et al*, 1994). It is a very useful method for studying behaviour directly; the correlation between what people say they do, and what they actually do, is often low, which makes both the interview and the questionnaire of limited value for behavioural studies. In contrast, attitudes cannot be reliably inferred from observing behaviour.

A further benefit of observation is that research participants can be observed in their natural environment, which provides a context in which to interpret their behaviour, as well as providing additional data. It is sometimes the case that people are not fully aware of their behaviour until it is observed by someone else; for example, that they are interacting with women clients more than men, or that they are constantly interrupting people of lower status than themselves in meetings.

Observation requires no effort on the part of research participants, and is particularly useful for studying people who are unwilling or unable to participate in more demanding methods. Like the interview and the questionnaire, observation may be highly structured or totally unstructured, and each can be placed somewhere along the following continuum:

Structured..........Semi-structured..........Unstructured

Structured observation

In structured observation, researchers decide exactly what to observe beforehand and will devise an observational schedule prior to the observations where the information can be categorized in a highly specific and systematic way. The environment in which the observations take place may be natural or may be manipulated in some way. For example, a physiotherapist who believes that cold therapy is more effective than ultrasound in reducing traumatic swelling following a ligament sprain, may test this hypothesis by observing the state of the swelling after treating one group of patients with cold therapy and another group with ultrasound over a period of time. This is an example of how observation is used within the experimental method (see Chapter 11). The point being made here is that observation can be an integral part of other research methods.

A highly structured approach can be used without manipulating the situation. For example an occupational therapy tutor, interested in comparing the teaching methods used in various colleges, may make very specific observations and record them in a highly structured way, but will not attempt to alter or manipulate the situation. The data obtained from structured observation is frequently suitable for statistical analysis (see Chapter 15).

Unstructured observation

In unstructured observation, researchers do not attempt to manipulate the situation they are investigating, instead they are interested in events as they occur naturally, and in the total situation rather than specific aspects of it. The data is usually recorded by means of notes, often written at the end of the day in the form of a diary. For example, a therapist interested in the interaction of clients being treated in groups, could observe a number of treatment groups over a period of weeks or months. The less structured the observation, the more inferences the researcher has to make, which can lead to poor reliability and validity. On the other hand, the information gained from unstructured observation is typically far richer than that obtained from a structured approach, which may render the data more valid. The researcher's agenda is, however, bound to influence what is extracted from the mass of perceptual data available. Video may help to validate the analysis as it can be checked by others.

Semi-structured observation

With semi-structured observation, researchers will be more concerned with some aspects of the situation than others, but they will also be keen to record any unusual or unique events as they arise, and will give such data considerable emphasis in their analysis. Therapists may use the semi-structured approach to observe the progress of disabled children in such activities as horse riding or swimming. Their main interest may be the children's physical development, but they are also likely to observe other interesting aspects, such as evidence of increased sociability or improved self-confidence. The data from semi-structured and unstructured observation is undertaken by means of content analysis (see Chapters 13 and 15).

How structured should the observation be?

Before deciding how structured or unstructured the observation should be, or indeed whether observation is the most appropriate method to use, researchers must be very clear about their research aims, questions or hypotheses.

A single observation may contain elements of the structured, semi-structured and unstructured approaches, and researchers may use different approaches at various phases of the same research project. Practical considerations will, of course, need to be taken into account. Observation, particularly if it is unstructured or semi-structured, tends to be very time-consuming and labour intensive though this will depend on the nature of each individual research project. If therapists need an entire year to observe the reactions of young children to hospitalization, this will obviously be very expensive and time-consuming, but if they manage to incorporate the study into their everyday work routine as paediatric therapists, then little expense will be incurred. Structured methods are linked to quantitative research, and semi-structured and unstructured methods are linked to qualitative research (see Chapter 15).

Stop and Think

Think of a research question that you would like to investigate by observation. You could, for example, observe the responses of therapists to reports of pain from male and female clients. Write down some of the ways in which your data would differ according to whether a structured or a less structured approach was used. What, if any, would be the benefit of combining a structured and a less structured approach in your research?

Researcher participation and participant awareness

As well as variations in the degree of structure within observational studies, they also vary in how far researchers involve themselves in the groups they are investigating. Furthermore, the research participants may or may not be aware that they are being observed. Every observation can therefore be placed on the following two continua:

Total researcher   No researcher
   participation................ participation

Maximum participant   No participant
   information.................... information

Thus the type of observation undertaken depends not only on the degree of structure, but also the extent to which the researcher participates in the group, and whether or not the research participants know they are being observed.

Uncontrolled non-participant observation

This type of observation is similar to that which we all engage in much of the time. Researchers do not attempt to control the situation in any way, and the research participants are not aware that they are being observed by a researcher. A researcher in this role has been referred to by Polgar and Thomas (1995) as a 'complete observer'.

A physiotherapist interested in the motor abilities of footballers, for example, may attend many football matches as a spectator in order to observe the footballers at play. The observations may be unstructured and undertaken in order to provide ideas before embarking on a research project, or they may be highly structured where an observational schedule is used to record specific events. Similarly, therapists may watch children at play to ascertain how well disabled children and non-disabled children interact; they will not be manipulating the situation in any way, and the children will be unaware of their presence.

Controlled non-participant observation

This type of observation is seen in experimental research. Researchers remain separate from the groups they are investigating while manipulating or controlling them in some way. For example, the staff of a centre for clients with challenging behaviour following head injury, may introduce various behavioural modification programmes and observe clients' behaviour to discover which programmes are the most effective. The example given above concerning the comparison between cold therapy and ultrasound also fits this category of observation.

Participant observation

In participant observation, researchers are members of the groups they are investigating. As mentioned above, the extent of their participation varies, as does the knowledge that the research participants have about the researcher's presence. A term used synonymously with participant observation is ethnography, which is described by Haralambos and Holborn as '... the study of a way of life' (1990: 740). Participant observation is the main method of ethnographic research but other methods such as interviewing and documentary research are also used (Banister et al, 1994).

Researchers may gain access to a group and openly observe it without taking much part in its activities. For example, a therapist interested in treatment techniques used to help people with mental health problems, could ask permission to observe other therapists at work. On the other hand, the researcher may have a secret agenda; for example, a sociologist may gain access to an occupational therapy department on the pretext that he or she is interested in pursuing occupational therapy as a career, when the purpose is really to investigate communication between therapists and their clients. Smith (1996) openly observed the working culture of physiotherapy assistants. Although Smith is a physiotherapist she distanced herself from that role by asking the assistants to regard her as a researcher and by not wearing a uniform.

If researchers are open about their roles it may be advantageous to use a video camera to record the observation. Researchers will then be able to observe the video repeatedly at their leisure and may ask other researchers to give their opinions or assist with the analysis. On the other hand permission to use a video camera may not be straightforward and research participants may react to it, rendering their behaviour unusual. The researcher may try to record everything, rather than being selective and information may be missed as video recorders have a restricted range (Foster, 1996).

It is sometimes possible to combine a genuine role with a concealed one. For example, therapists interested in the dynamics of inter-disciplinary team meetings may contribute to the meetings in their role as therapists, but at the same time study the dynamics of the group in their secret role as researcher. In this case the therapists could be described as 'insider' researchers because of their personal involvement in the area being investigated. It is sometimes said that 'insider' researchers lack objectivity because of their close involvement with the research topic but, on the other hand, they have the advantage of understanding the issues in depth which may enable them to make more valid and subtle interpretations. Talking of research on disabled people Moore claims that:

> Trying to maintain distance as an observer ... does not ensure that a truer image of events and practices will be assembled but can yield restrained and possibly corrupt research outputs. (1998: 34)

Much has been learned from feminist research which has shown that even the most 'objective' research has been shaped by the perceptions and experiences of men, and that 'insider' research can be more valid.

The main advantage of honesty and openness in observational research, is that researchers are free to ask questions and to observe and record the information they receive openly. The main disadvantage is that they are likely to alter unwittingly the behaviour of the people they are observing. If a group of patients engaged in circuit training is being observed by a researcher, for example, they may try extra hard to succeed, making their behaviour atypical. This problem can be overcome to a large extent if researchers stay with the group for a considerable period of time, as research participants will become less affected by their presence. It can be argued, however, that provided research participants are certain of confidentiality, they may be more honest when observed and interviewed by a stranger, than by a peer or manager, because what they say and do will have no personal consequences for them.

The complete participant

In this type of observation, which has been used extensively by anthropologists, researchers become full members of the communities under investigation and their roles are completely concealed; for example, a person wishing to study the day-to-day work of physiotherapists may gain employment as a physiotherapy assistant, or even go to the lengths of becoming a physiotherapist purely for research purposes. Similarly an occupational therapist wishing to observe the activities of a self-help group, may pose as a genuine member. Erving Goffman became an orderly in a psychiatric hospital to provide data for his famous book *Asylums* (Goffman, 1961), Rosenhan (1973) feigned mental illness and became a patient to investigate how patients in psychiatric institutions are treated by staff, and Holmes and Johnson (1988) gained employment as care assistants in a variety of old people's homes to investigate the practices within them.

There are many problems with the role of participant observer, especially if the role is covert. The deception and pretense which is often involved in carrying the research through is not easy to cope with and can cause the researcher a great deal of anxiety, especially as successful observation is dependent on good, co-operative relationships with the group under investigation. The researcher may come to feel great respect and friendship for people in the group and yet must continue to deceive them. It is unlikely that covert research by undergraduate therapists would be approved by ethics committees, as greater protection is now given to potential research participants.

There are various problems for researchers who become complete participants. First, their own behaviour may influence the activities of the groups they are investigating; therapists observing the dynamics of multidisciplinary team meetings, for example, may consciously or subconsciously influence the proceedings of the group by their own behaviour. Second, it may be very difficult for a researcher of dissimilar background or culture to those being observed, to understand their behaviour, or to draw valid inferences from it. This may occur if therapists are observing clients from an ethnic minority group. Despite these problems, if people are observed in a natural environment over a period of time, the data often proves more valid than that obtained from a structured approach. Researchers may, for example, gain a great deal of information about the micro-culture of therapy departments which would be difficult to access through interviews or questionnaires, because research partici-pants may be unaware of the issues or unable to articulate them fully.

Polgar and Thomas (1995) use the following terms to describe the role of the researcher engaged in observation:

- 'Complete observer' where researchers have no involve-ment at all in the groups they are investigating.
- 'Observer as participant' where researchers interact freely with members of the group but make no effort to become members themselves.
- 'Participant as observer' where researchers participate fully in the group but disclose their purpose and identity.
- 'Complete participant' where researchers are full members of the groups they are investigating and where their roles are concealed.

Ethical considerations

Stop and Think
Imagine that you are involved in a covert research project either in your place of work or your college. Make a list of the ethical implications you would face. Could you justify your actions? If so, how?

There are various ethical issues which must be examined very carefully by anyone considering the use of observation in research, especially if it is covert. Many groups who have been the subject of observational research, for example homeless people and prisoners, have lacked the power to complain about such intrusions.

Researchers may witness events which they find disturbing, or with which they disapprove. If, for example, researchers witness the ill-treatment of clients, they will be faced with the dilemma of whether to report it or whether to continue their observations in order to gather evidence and document the ill-treatment later. If researchers give voice to their views they may antagonize the group they are investigating, resulting in loss of co-operation.

Many people disapprove of covert methods, so researchers must be prepared for criticism, or even worse consequences, if they publish their work. It is also possible that research of this type could be damaging to the therapy professions, because if it became widespread practice, people might become highly suspicious of therapists and no longer trust them to undertake research.

Others believe that covert methods can be justified if the benefits are likely to outweigh any damage that is done, or if the groups being investigated are known to be devious themselves. Considerable data on unjust discrimination, for example, has been gathered by means of covert methods, and it is doubtful whether the data could have been collected in any other way. Graham (1990), for example, uncovered considerable discrimination against physically disabled people in the employment market by writing letters to employers by fictitious disabled and non-disabled people with the same qualifications. (See Chapter 3 for further discussion of ethical issues.)

Recording observational data

Structured observation

Researchers who wish to undertake a structured or semi-structured observation will need to devise an observational schedule prior to the observation. Before doing so it can be helpful to examine schedules compiled by those who have conducted similar research. Such schedules may occasionally suffice or, more usually, may serve as a framework for the design of a new one.

When constructing observational schedules each category of behaviour to be recorded must be defined very carefully; it is not enough for researchers to indicate that they will be observing 'aggression' or 'improvement' without defining what these concepts mean in terms of behaviour. Each category must be mutually exclusive and exhaustive. This means that it should only be possible to assign each observed behavioural event to one category, and that it should be possible to categorize every piece of relevant behaviour observed.

A simple observational schedule for recording the behaviour of six patients is shown in figure 12.1.

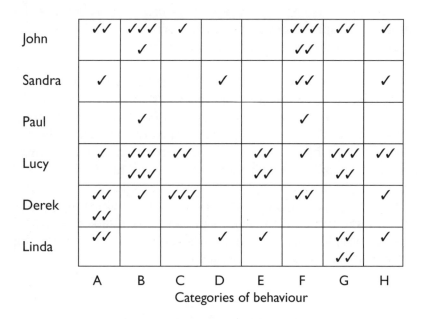

	A	B	C	D	E	F	G	H
John	✓✓	✓✓✓ ✓	✓			✓✓✓ ✓✓	✓✓	✓
Sandra	✓			✓		✓✓		✓
Paul		✓				✓		
Lucy	✓	✓✓✓ ✓✓✓	✓✓		✓✓ ✓✓	✓	✓✓✓ ✓✓	✓✓
Derek	✓✓ ✓✓	✓	✓✓✓			✓✓		✓
Linda	✓✓			✓	✓		✓✓ ✓✓	✓

Categories of behaviour

Figure 12.1 A simple observational schedule

It is also possible to observe and record the interaction of groups. This is illustrated in Figure 12.2.

Sturgens (1999) observed children undergoing an assessment in occupational therapy and devised a list of their behaviours which were recorded on a grid. These behaviours included 'hesitating', 'ridiculing the question' and 'giving needlessly long answers'. As well as being useful in modifying the assessment tool, it placed the assessment scores into a broader interpretive framework where the child's personality and affective state could be taken into account.

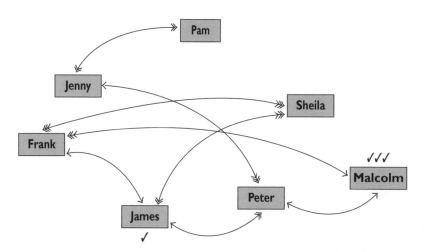

Figure 12.2 An observational schedule showing the interaction of a group. Arrows indicate communication between individuals; ticks indicate communication with the whole group

Stop and Think
Devise a simple observational schedule to gather data for a small research project of your choice. You may, for example, decide to observe the different behaviours of a group of clients in an ante-natal session. Explain why this method of structured observation is particularly useful and how the knowledge you gain may be used in therapy.

Even with highly systematic methods of observation we always interpret what we see and hear from our own perspective, which can give rise to personal bias. To minimize this effect, structured observations can be undertaken by several researchers after a period of training. Any disagreements they have can be discussed and the schedule adjusted and refined until the level of agreement among them is high. This type of training improves reliability, but has the disadvantage that the perceptions of particularly insightful researchers may be lost, with a consequent reduction of validity. The data from structured observations is analysed by means of statistics (see Chapter 15).

Semi-structured and unstructured observation

The data from semi-structured and unstructured observations are likely to be in the form of hand-written notes. These notes may include descriptions of events, theoretical analyses, details of methods, and the researcher's own feelings and perceptions. If possible, events observed should be recorded immediately to minimize errors and distortions of memory. Information from structured and semi-structured observation is analysed by means of content analysis and other qualitative methods (see Chapters 13 and 15).

Sampling

Deciding which situations to observe, and when and where the observations should take place, will depend on the particular research questions posed, as well as various practical considerations such as time constraints and available resources. If researchers wish to obtain representative samples of behaviour, it is better for them to observe for short periods on many occasions, than to observe for long periods on a few occasions. If they wish to generalize their data beyond the particular situation they are observing, then a variety of settings must be used. If, on the other hand, researchers want to gain a detailed understanding of the events they are observing, then it would be better for them to observe for long periods on a few occasions.

Time sampling

A systematic time sampling technique can be used to gather data. While observing a particular client, for example, his or her behaviour could be recorded on the observational schedule every ten seconds. Rather than being systematic, the time intervals themselves can be randomly selected. A major disadvantage of time sampling is that important events which occur infrequently may never be observed. In addition the data tends to lack continuity; it is often unclear how events are related, especially if the time intervals between observations are long. The context in which the behaviour takes place is also partially lost. The researcher may, for example, record the challenging behaviour of a patient being observed without fully understanding the events which precipitated it.

Event sampling

In event sampling, specific events are recorded as they occur. For example, a therapist may observe a group of older people in a residential home to see how often they engage in certain types of behaviour such as walking, talking to each other, or reading the newspaper. Every time the event occurs the therapist can record it. This technique is particularly useful for recording unusual or infrequent incidents, it also enables the researcher to record complete episodes from beginning to end. Time sampling and event sampling can be combined if advantages are to be gained by doing so. (For further details of sampling, see Chapter 7).

Stop and Think
Go back to your last activity where you devised an observational schedule. Consider how you would sample the behaviour and explain the choices you have made.

The pilot study

Before an observational study is undertaken, it is important to carry out a few observations to test the observational schedule and eliminate any problems that may have been overlooked. For example, one category may be difficult to distinguish from another, or an important aspect of behaviour may appear to fit nowhere on the schedule. The people observed in the pilot study should be as similar to the 'real' research participants as possible.

Trace measures

The use of trace measures to gather evidence is an example of unobtrusive, observational research, which can be defined as research where little or no contact takes place between the researcher and the research participants. Trace measures are rarely used in isolation unless there is no alternative; more commonly they are employed in conjunction with other methods, such as questionnaires or interviews. They may also be used during the early stages of the research process when the researcher is attempting to generate research questions or hypotheses.

Trace measures are of two types:

1. Erosion measures – the selective wearing of surfaces and objects.
2. Accretion measures – the materials left behind by a population, for example litter, graffiti, tools, tombstones etc.

We are all familiar with trace measures and how they provide us with information and evidence of what is happening in our daily lives. Our suspicion may, for example, be aroused by some unexplained footprints on the garden, we may notice that the cat has taken to sleeping on the bed in our absence, or that the carpet or lawn is wearing thin in a particular place; we also judge and value the worth of objects by how well they wear. Archaeologists are almost totally dependent on trace measures in their research, and the police make great use of them in their investigations, for example the analysis of DNA samples and fingerprints which may be left behind at the scene of a crime.

Physical traces of various kinds can provide valuable data to researchers with diverse interests. The wear and tear of the grass under each item in a children's playground may give some indication of their relative use, and the degree of wear and tear on library books may indicate their popularity. Graffiti has been used as a rich source of data among social scientists and historians.

A therapist interested in the effects of an anti-smoking campaign in the hospital where he or she works could compare the number of cigarette ends left at the end of the day before, during and after the campaign. Similarly a therapist studying the effects of environmental change on long-stay clients with mental health problems could use measures of litter, cigarette ends and graffiti as indicators of their morale. A therapist interested in discovering which toys a group of disabled children play with most could gain some information by noting the wear and tear of the toys over a period of time, and therapists studying the gait of people with various lower limb impairments could observe the wear and tear of their shoes. Domholdt states that evidence such as this '... contributes to the breadth and depth of information collected by the qualitative researcher' (2000: 164).

The advantages and limitations of trace measures in research

The main advantage of using trace measures in research is that there is no contact between the researcher and the research participants. As noted in earlier chapters, this contact can give rise to effects which threaten the validity of the research; for example the research participant may be anxious or keen to create a good impression, and the researcher may unwittingly influence the behaviour of research participants, or be unduly influenced by their accents or appearance.

Despite this important advantage, there are a number of limitations which must be borne in mind when using trace measures in research. The amount of litter or graffiti present could be highly significant but may, alternatively, merely reflect the number of cleaners employed and how hard they work. The researcher has little control over the situation when using trace measures, and has limited information about the population under investigation. The analysis is therefore likely to be partial, and further sources of data are usually needed before accurate interpretations can be made.

Conclusion

Observation is an ideal method for gathering information about behaviour, although it is not suitable for studying very intimate behaviour. Observation is a suitable method for use in a wide variety of health care settings, but because of the covert nature of some observational approaches, it is fraught with a greater number of ethical issues than many other research methods.

The use of documents in research

Documentary research refers to the collation and analysis of written documents such as official reports, textbooks, newspapers and novels; and visual and auditory material, such as films, speeches and radio and television programmes. Pamphlets, time-tables, maps, posters, paintings and photographs can all be used in documentary research, as well as data stored on computer (Denscombe, 1998; Hammell *et al*, 2000). Documentary research may be used as a research method in its own right, for example when analysing written documents and photographs to conduct historical research; as one of several methods in a multi-method approach, for example when using video clips prior to a group interview: and as an integral aspect of another method, for example the analysis of interview transcripts or diaries written by research participants.

For ease of description it is customary to divide documents into primary and secondary sources. Primary data exist before the research project begins; examples include government statistics and official reports. It is very important that primary sources which are cited in research reports are correctly referenced so that readers are able to find them if they wish. Secondary sources of data are produced by the people who gather the information or by the research participants themselves, for example the field notes kept by a researcher involved in participant observations, the transcripts of semi-structured interviews and the diaries kept by research participants (Finnegan, 1996).

Scott (1990) has categorized primary documents into four main types:

1. Closed documents – those to which researchers have no access, such as certain government reports.
2. Semi-closed documents – those with restricted access, which may be open to researchers following negotiation.
3. Open-archival documents – those which are available and are situated in archives.
4. Open-published documents – those which are published and readily available in shops and libraries.

The first class of document is likely to be covered by the Official Secrets Act and the second by the Data Protection Act. The Data Protection Act, which came into force in 1984, controls and restricts the use of some personal data. Researchers who wish to use such data must be registered under the terms of the Act. Guidelines for researchers are available from the Data Protection Register.

Stop and Think
Imagine that you are about to use a variety of documents to investigate the occupational therapy or physiotherapy treatment of paraplegia over the past thirty years. How much confidence would you have in the documents? Would you need to ask yourself any questions before accepting that the documents are valid?

When analysing any document researchers need to ask themselves the following questions:

How representative is the document?
Existing documents are often unrepresentative of others of their type. Some documents are deliberately destroyed, and those which are housed in archives are generally selected from a far

larger sample. Documents, such as letters and diaries, from as little as 150 years ago, would only have been written by educated people, while biographies focus almost exclusively on the famous and exceptional. Which statistics are considered worthy of collection is also important; there is far more official information on poor people in our society than rich people, because the former are subject to greater scrutiny and assessment by professionals and the state. In contrast, the voice of oppressed and minority groups, such as people with learning difficulties, are often absent in official documents as though their existence is of little, if any, importance (Atkinson *et al*, 1997). It does not necessarily matter to researchers that documents are unrepresentative, but it is vital that researchers (and those who read the research) know that they are in order to reach valid conclusions.

Is the document authentic?
This issue is unlikely to be of great significance to therapists undertaking documentary research, but it can be vital to historians when, for example, an old document or a lost painting is discovered. It is also an issue of central concern to the police as they attempt to ascertain whether a letter is genuine or a forgery, or whether a sample of handwriting is that of a wanted criminal. For therapists the issue could become important in cases of litigation, where the authenticity of a medical record may be in doubt.

Is the document credible?
It is important that researchers discover just how accurate the document is. In order to ascertain the credibility of a document, it is necessary to have some information about the author, and to know why the document was written. Was it written to show the author in the best possible light? Was it for purposes of propaganda? Was it written under someone else's direction? In some research carried out by French (1996) on the memories of eight visually impaired women who, as children, had attended a special residential school, the account given by the women was in sharp contrast to that given in the official annual reports. This is illustrated in the following extracts:

The care of the partially sighted places a special responsibility on the matrons and domestic staff, the warm thanks of the governors are due to them for the selfless way in which they fulfil their duties. (Annual Report, 1959–60: 16)

Even as nippers we were made to stand facing the wall for hours at a time. Quite regularly we would get the ruler across the legs very hard. There might be no sweets for weeks or we were sent to bed without tea. Quite often privileges like play time were missed, instead we would have to stand in the corner very straight. (French, 1996: 30)

The interview data throw doubt upon the credibility of the official reports which, in this case, was one of the aims of undertaking the research.

What does the document mean?
Researchers need to make every effort to understand the meaning of documents. To achieve this it is necessary to comprehend the conditions under which they were produced. As Scott states, 'The particular way in which a concept was defined and applied in practice changes over time and from place to place.' (1990: 8) Ways of recording data vary, and are based on underlying assumptions and perceptions which are shaped by political, cultural and ideological factors. The terminology and classification of illness, for example, has changed over the years and differs from country to country; in Britain old age was classified as a cause of death until the beginning of the twentieth century, and scarlet fever and diphtheria were classified as one disease until 1855.

In a very real sense data are not collected but created. Whether or not a death is classified as suicide, for example, will depend on the ideas and perceptions of coroners at a given point in history, which will, in turn, be influenced by the society in which they live. The construction of meaning is a circular process with official meanings shaping everyday meanings and vice versa. It is also a political process as certain groups have the power to impose their meanings on others. As May states:

... what people decide to record, to leave in or take out, is itself informed by decisions which relate to the social, political and economic environment of which they are a part. (1997: 176)

There is often little consensus, however, with agencies tending to define such concepts as 'unemployment', 'old age', 'health' and 'disability' in diverse ways. It is essential that therapists attempt to grasp the underlying meaning of any document they use in research.

It can be seen from this discussion of meaning that documents can be used for two distinct, but inter-related, purposes in research. They may be used as sources of information, for example when a therapist consults a statistical report to discover the extent of industrial accidents; or they may, of themselves, be the focus of study, for example when a therapist investigates their creation in order to understand the assumptions and perceptions underlying a particular illness at a given time. The official documentation associated with mental handicap hospitals, for example, can give insight into the thinking behind the incarceration of large numbers of people in institutions (Barclay, 1999).

Stop and Think
Think back to activity 1 where you investigated the treatment of paraplegia over a thirty-year period by the use of various documents. Think of at least three ways in which this information could be measured and analysed.

Content analysis

Documents are analysed by means of content analysis. When undertaking a content analysis, it is necessary to formulate the research question, and then to define and select the documents to be analysed. For example, a therapist wishing to investigate whether or not his or her profession has become more involved in research activity over the years, may decide to analyse the profession's major journal to discover whether the number of research articles written by therapists has increased, how much discussion of research exists on the letter page and how many courses on research are advertised. It will not be possible for the therapist to analyse every journal, of course, so sampling will be necessary. Perhaps the therapist will concentrate on the last ten years of journals and take a random sample of five from each.

Measuring the data

The data contained within documents and audio and visual material, may be measured in terms of their structure and their content.

Quantity (time and space): This may include the measurement of column inches, the size of print, or the length of a speech or radio programme. Colour and the location of items or photographs on a page can also be measured. Such measures can indicate the importance of a topic, or the status of the person involved with presenting it. For example, a great deal of 'column inches' in newspapers has been devoted to the topic of AIDS, and the length of time a person is given to make a speech can be an indication of his or her status. Black and white images are often associated with topics deemed to be tragic, such as disability.

Frequency: The number of times a specific item, such as a word, image or theme, occurs in a document can be counted. Frequency counts can give an indication of underlying perceptions and assumptions, and may be a useful indicator of the importance of a topic. Reynolds (1996a) counted the number of words physiotherapy students and occupational therapy students used in their essays in relation to specific communication skills. It was found in this analysis that occupational therapy students placed more emphasis than physiotherapy students on patients' emotional and relationship needs. Frequency counts can also be used to ascertain the authenticity of a document, as people are individualistic in the words and phrases they use. This type of analysis can often be undertaken using a computer.

Morris and Morris (1995) analysed images of physiotherapists in advertisements in 32 editions of *Physiotherapy* from January 1992 to August 1995. Forty per cent of the images were male whereas, in reality, only 7% of physiotherapists were male at this time. All of the images depicted Caucasians and 98% were judged to be under 35 years of age. The authors conclude that:

> ... the young and white image portrayed probably conforms to the current ageist and racist views prevalent within society and within health care advertising. (1995: 294)

Amitstead (1997) studied initial non-attendance rates of physiotherapy treatment by scrutinizing patients' referral cards. She found that men were less likely to keep their initial appointment than women and that people between the ages of 21 and 50 were least likely to attend. Those who were referred by a GP were less likely to attend than those who were referred by a consultant.

Intensity: This is a rather more subjective measure as it depends on the researcher making judgements, although detailed guidelines may be devised. For example, a therapist analysing a report concerning disabled people may classify words or ideas as 'positive', 'neutral' or 'negative', or a therapist reading the results of various case studies concerning the effectiveness of a behaviour modification programme may classify them as 'good', 'fair' or 'poor'. Tutors marking examination scripts are also required to make judgements of this type.

With a quantitative content analysis the researcher needs to construct a coding frame where units of information, for example male images of physiotherapists, can be allocated. It is important that these categories are mutually exclusive, that is a unit of information can only be allocated to one category, and that they are exhaustive, that is they accommodate all the information of interest to the researcher. The data can then be analysed with the use of descriptive statistics such as histograms and pie charts (see Chapter 15). Content analysis may be qualitative as well as quantitative where, for example, the researcher categorizes the data into major themes or writes case studies from the data. Qualitative approaches to the analysis of documents is discussed in Chapter 15.

Documents used in documentary research

> **Stop and Think**
> What documents would you as a therapist consider using in research? Would there be any problems in accessing such documents?

Any document, or visual or auditory material, is suitable for analysis by researchers. Below are some of the materials which may be used in documentary research by therapists.

Case notes and medical files

Case notes and medical files may be used by therapists in a number of ways in research and in clinical audit. Attendance patterns or the language that therapists use when describing patients or their symptoms may, for example, be analysed. Treatment trends may be examined, as well as the differential ways in which records may be kept by different professionals. Access to records for research purposes may not, however, be straightforward because of issues of confidentiality. It is likely that permission will need to be sought from an ethics committee.

Autobiographies and biographies

Autobiographies and biographies can provide an extremely rich source of data for researchers, including details of unusual personal experiences. They have the advantage of taking the individual's viewpoint into account and can provide an element of human interest which other research methods may lack. Autobiographies may also give the researcher ideas for the formulation of research questions and hypotheses. This is important as professional meanings of a concept, such as illness, may be limited, leading to bias in the type of research undertaken and the type of knowledge produced.

When a large number of autobiographies on the same theme have been written, it is possible to make tentative generalizations which a single autobiography would not allow. A therapist interested in the coping strategies of people with spinal cord injuries, for example, may decide to read ten autobiographies written by people with spinal cord injuries and carry out a content analysis (see Chapter 15). Although each autobiography will give a highly personal account, the researcher may notice a few dominant coping strategies which are employed, or alternatively, may be struck by their diversity, or the way they change over time.

The use of autobiographies and biographies in research does have limitations. For example, the authors are likely to omit various aspects of their stories which might place them in a poor light or cause offence or upset to others. Memories may be distorted, and it may be necessary to emphasize unusual or sensational aspects of the person's life in order for the book to be published, leading to bias in the information presented and, possibly, a blurring of fact and fiction. As Hammersley and Atkinson state:

> Authors will have interests in presenting themselves in a (usually) favourable light; they may also have axes to grind, scores to settle, or excuses and justifications to make. (1983: 130)

The information in biographies is also likely to be distorted, in fact the author's motive in writing the biography may be to portray the person in the best possible light, perhaps in response to other biographies which have sought to discredit the individual concerned.

People who write autobiographies cannot be described as 'ordinary', most being either famous or having some unusual experiences to relate. Furthermore it is simply not the sort of activity that most of us engage in, even if we do feel we have something interesting to say. The task of writing an autobiography is also very time-consuming and demands considerable literacy skills.

Diaries

There are various ways in which diaries may be used in research. If personal diaries are analysed, the advantages and disadvantages are similar to those of the autobiography and biography. If diarists do not intend their material to be read, they may give a more honest account, although dishonesty and self-justification may still be present. Diaries have the advantage that they are usually written close in time to the events they record and thus suffer less than autobiographies and biographies from retrospective effects; neither are they distorted by the work of editors. Some diaries give very factual information, for example appointment diaries and log books.

Diaries can be useful in the study of private behaviour where observation is inappropriate or impractical. For example, a researcher may ask a group of people who are trying to lose weight to keep a diary recording the amount and content of the food they eat, and the type and amount of exercise they take. Alternatively research participants, such as therapists, may be asked to record critical incidents or problems which they encounter at work. As with the questionnaire and interview, great care must be taken with the wording of questions, though sometimes participants may simply be asked to tick boxes in a grid every time a particular event occurs. Whatever the task, researchers must be sure that participants are able to carry it out and that they have the time and motivation to do so.

A disadvantage of this method is that researchers are obliged to rely on the motivation and accuracy of research participants in keeping the diary. The fact that they have been asked to do so can also have an effect on their behaviour, thereby distorting the data. For example, if a researcher is interested in analysing a person's behaviour when trying to lose weight this may, in itself, be sufficient to stimulate that person to lose weight. Used in this way, the diary cannot, therefore, be regarded as a truly unobtrusive research tool.

Researchers may also use diaries to collect their own data, this is common practice among those engaged in participant observation.

Newspapers and magazines

Newspapers and magazines provide a vast source of data on practically every topic, including health, illness and disability. However, they tend to concentrate on topical issues and there is frequent distortion as information is cut and rearranged; in addition, many national newspapers reflect a particular political angle. Such data would, however, be invaluable to therapists wishing to investigate lay concepts of health or illness. For example, they could analyse accounts of AIDS or cancer given in various popular newspapers and magazines, and perhaps compare these accounts with those in medical textbooks.

Professional journals

Although professional journals tend to be seen as objective and scientific, researchers need to realize that many of the problems associated with newspapers and magazines apply equally to journals. Professional bodies are politically sensitive organizations which can result in the rejection of papers which are critical of the profession, or which oppose an established view, regardless of their relevance, importance or standard. There may be a tendency to concentrate on a particular type of research, or only to publish statistically significant findings (French, 1993). All of this will shape the knowledge produced in a particular direction.

Professional journals can, however, be of tremendous use to therapists undertaking documentary research. For example, by undertaking a content analysis of the last five years of a professional journal, it may be possible to find significant trends, for instance in the attitudes of therapists towards psychiatric illness, the use of a particular treatment approach, or the language used to describe a group of people such as those with learning difficulties.

Essays

Neville and French (1991) asked physiotherapy students to write short essays on what they considered to be a 'good' and a 'poor' clinical experience. Therapists could use this method of research for any number of projects. For example they could ask disabled children to write about their feelings concerning therapy, or the difficulties they experience in mainstream school. The method does, however, favour articulate and literate people, and the content may be dramatized in an attempt to write a 'good' essay.

Official statistics

Official statistics are collected by the state and its agencies. Examples include the census, which is a questionnaire sent to every household every ten years, and the registration of births, deaths and marriages. There is a great deal of statistical data available concerning health, illness and disability. Many official statistics are published annually and are readily available in libraries and book shops. Examples of these are *Social Trends* and *Regional Trends*. Unofficial statistics, perhaps those routinely gathered in therapy departments, can also be used in research.

It is important to comprehend the terminology when using official statistics. Many terms, for example 'illness' and 'disability', are difficult to define and may change over time and from place to place, making temporal and cross-cultural comparisons difficult. People are also sensitive to the social and political nuances of the time when responding to questionnaires. They may, for example, respond differently to questions concerning ethnicity now than they would have done ten years ago, even though the question wording, and their attitudes, remain the same.

Official statistics provide a wealth of data but there is a great danger of viewing them as more reliable and objective than they really are. Statistics can be manipulated for political purposes, so it is important to ascertain who sponsored the study and what the research was for. If data produced is perceived to be politically damaging, it may be rejected or parts of it omitted or minimized. In addition, official statistics rarely reflect reality, for example the amount of crime reported is unlikely to tally with the amount of crime committed, and the amount of illness reported is an underestimation of the amount of illness which exists (French, 1997). It is advisable that therapists using official statistics in their research should try to discover the sampling techniques used as well as the response rate obtained. If possible the recording instrument (for example a questionnaire) should also be scrutinized to determine its reliability and validity. As Denscombe states:

> Certain types of official statistics will, to all intents and purposes, provide an objective picture of reality. Unfortunately, the same cannot be said for certain other types of official statistics. When politicians debate the accuracy of unemployment figures or the significance of particular national economic figures, there is clearly room for some doubt and controversy about the objectivity, the accuracy, the completeness and the relevance of some official statistics. (1998: 164)

Official documents which are gathered within therapy departments may also be used in research, such as the minutes of meetings, policy documents and records of accidents.

Stop and Think
Choose any two of the above types of documents (or others from your own choice) and devise a small research project of interest to you which uses these documents as a source of data. What do you consider to be the advantages and disadvantages of using documentary evidence in your research project?

Advantages and disadvantages of documentary research

Documentary research has a number of distinct advantages when compared with some other research methods. It is relatively economical and largely unobtrusive, and enables researchers to analyse large amounts of high quality data which already exists. No other organization but government has the resources or the power to undertake such wide-ranging surveys as the census, and it is only surveys such as this which permit comparisons and trends of large populations over time and across cultures, or provide sufficient data for large scale quantitative analyses of minority groups.

Documentary data may overcome various ethical issues. For example, it may be possible to analyse people's reactions to a disaster without involving them in any way (for example through letters, articles and statistics on post-traumatic stress syndrome) and there may be little need to go through an ethics committee. Documentary research is certainly not, however, divorced from ethical issues. As Homan points out:

> Data may be collected for an initial purpose which subjects regard as worthy, translated into statistical form and so stored, and then used for another purpose by a secondary analyst. (1991: 90)

It must also be emphasized that patients' clinical notes and their work (for example art work from a therapy session) may need clearance by an ethics committee. Similarly the use of television programmes and autobiographies by researchers may need permission from authors, broadcasting companies and publishers.

The disadvantages of documentary research are that it can be isolating and time-consuming to undertake, and is restricted to topics which have been spoken and written about. The representativeness, credibility, authenticity and meaning of the documents is frequently in doubt and the information may be incomplete.

Conclusion

Documentary research is not, perhaps, the first method that would spring to the minds of therapists wanting to undertake research. It can, however, be very valuable either as the sole research method, as one among others in a multi-method approach, or as an integral part of other methods. It provides therapists with a vast array of ready made, and often high quality, data, and can be invaluable in answering various research questions. It provides an efficient and cost-effective way for therapists to engage in research. Information may, however, be incomplete or may be insufficiently tailored to the researcher's aims.

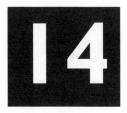

The case study

Case studies provide a detailed description and analysis of a single event, group, institution or person within its own social context. A case study can involve a unit as small as an individual or as large as an entire community. It provides an opportunity to carry out an in-depth study of a particular individual, situation or event. The case study can provide preliminary data before the researcher embarks on a full-scale study, perhaps to accumulate knowledge before devising research tools such as a questionnaire. Case studies can also be useful as the means of generating hypotheses and research questions. Conversely, the case study can be used after a large scale project is completed in an attempt to explain unusual or unexpected findings. The case study can, however, be used as a research strategy in its own right.

The case study was by far the most popular mode of clinical investigation during the first half of the twentieth century, but it fell into disrepute on the grounds of being unscientific. However, it is uniquely suited to the production of certain types of knowledge, and in particular to the development of theory. This realization, together with a growing number of critiques of 'scientific' and 'objective' research (see Bryman, 1988; Banister *et al*, 1994) has rendered the case study acceptable again.

The case study enables researchers to investigate particular individuals or situations intensively over time. Case studies produce data which would be missed or remain hidden in large scale studies. Denscombe states that:

> What a case study can do that a survey normally cannot is to study things in detail. When a researcher takes the strategic decision to devote all his or her effort to researching just one instance, there is obviously far greater opportunity to delve into things in more detail and discover things that might not have been apparent through more superficial research. (1998: 30–31)

The case study is an holistic research approach which can unravel the complexities of a situation. It enables the researcher to discover the interrelationships among various factors and the processes which occur to bring about varying outcomes. Case studies focus on real life events that happen naturally. Stake asserts that '... the distinctive need for case studies arises out of the desire to understand complex social phenomena' (1995: 3) and Bell believes that a successful case study will '... illustrate relationships, micropolitical issues and patterns of influences in a particular context' (1999: 12).

Any method or combination of methods can be used in case study research including interviews, observation and the use of documentary evidence (Yin, 1994; Descombe, 1998). The case study can be regarded, therefore, as a research approach or strategy rather than a research method. Both quantitative and qualitative methods are appropriate; for example the researcher may carry out a series of highly structured observations of an individual, but also undertake an open-ended interview. Existing, standardized tests can also be used.

The case study can be carried out during or after an event, the latter often referred to as a case history. Frequently a number of case studies are combined, in order to find common themes or differences in outcome (Seale and Barnard, 1998). An example of a research study which used multiple case studies is that by Foster (1987) who investigated the process of institutionalization and deinstitutionalization of people with severe learning difficulties by means of observation, interviews and the analysis of official documents. She found that institutionalization and deinstitutionalization were socially and politically constructed.

The findings from a case study can also be mapped against the findings of other studies within the research literature. A study of the working lives of visually impaired physiotherapists (French, 2000) for example, revealed that the barriers they face at work are similar to those of other visually impaired employees.

Case studies can be carried out to explore therapy interventions in more depth. Reynolds (1996b), for example, conducting a case study on a woman with moderate depression to explore the contribution of physical activity to affective and cognitive expression during counselling.

Case studies need to be distinguished from case reports although the two terms are often used interchangeably. Case studies provide a detailed and systematic description and analysis of a phenomena within its own social and environmental context whereas case reports, within therapy, are more descriptive and focus on clinical practice. Case reports are usually dismissed as 'not research' although Domholdt (2000) and others take issue with this, believing that they can contribute to both theory and practice.

Stop and Think

Think of a client at your place of work, or on a recent clinical visit, that you consider to be a suitable participant for case study research. What would be the value of conducting a case study on this client? List at least three reasons for choosing the case study as your research strategy.

Advantages of the case study approach

The case study is an excellent approach if the researcher requires a detailed understanding of a specific person or event. The aim may be to help plan an effective treatment programme or to develop a theoretical concept; in the former the results may be put into practice immediately. Stake asserts that 'We are interested in it (the case) not because by studying it we learn about other cases ... but because we need to learn about that particular case' (1995: 3). The case can, therefore, be studied for its own sake and not to make generalizations. Although the knowledge produced relates to a particular person, group or situation, it may, nonetheless, be helpful to other people. With regard to therapists, Bailey states that 'Most of us have at least one client whose progress and style of learning could benefit others' (1991: 63).

The data produced in case studies can cast doubt on 'taken-for-granted' knowledge or theoretical assumptions. As Arksey and Knight state '... even a single case study can call into question the assumptions of a theory' (1999: 59). At the very least broad generalizations may be modified by a single case study. This is illustrated in the following example.

Ponsford and French (1989) carried out a case study of a man who had learned to drive, and who earned his living as a driver, despite severe athetoid cerebral palsy affecting all his limbs. The stimulus to undertake this study was provided when the man, Mr. T, drove a friend of his to a centre where driving assessment and instruction are given to disabled people. The staff at the centre (including one of the researchers), seeing Mr. T and believing him to be a client, immediately felt pessimistic and thought it highly unlikely that he would be able to drive.

The case study included a detailed physical examination of Mr. T, a structured observation of his driving skills, and several short in-depth interviews which were necessary as Mr. T has severe dysarthria. Mr. T's driving skills, though different from those of non-disabled people, were found to be satisfactory in every respect which threw doubt on the assumptions of the staff that people with severe athetosis cannot drive.

The interviews with Mr. T revealed that no driving instructor had been prepared to teach him and that he had received instruction over several years from an elderly neighbour who had plenty of time. The ability to drive is a highly important factor in the quality of Mr. T's life for, as well as requiring the skill in his job, he is also a single parent and is unable to use public transport. Research methods which concentrate on groups of people may miss unusual instances such as this. Case studies, such as that of Mr. T, can help us to understand in depth the skills that individuals acquire to deal with the difficulties they encounter.

The case study is one of the few research approaches available to investigate unique or unusual events, for example rare syndromes and medical conditions, such as congenital indifference to pain, or unusual social situations. A famous case study is that described by Koluchova (1976), concerning twin boys who were kept isolated and were almost totally neglected from the age of eighteen months to seven years. The subsequent rapid improvement in their abilities, after they were fostered in a loving home, threw doubt on assumptions concerning the prognosis of seriously deprived and neglected children. It is not, however, a requirement that the topic of case studies be unusual or sensational; indeed a criticism of case study research is that it has tended to concentrate on sensational issues to the exclusion of the less dramatic.

Boyd Boonyauiroj (1996) carried out a case study concerning a very common situation, a physiotherapist returning to work after a career break. The physiotherapist, Martin, kept a diary from the first day of his employment to the end of the fifth month. After this period he also responded in writing to 15 written questions including, 'Out of everything, what did you find the hardest?' and 'if you gave advice to facilitate those who hire someone like you, what would you say?' He was also asked to rate his self-confidence over the five-month period.

A content analysis of his diary and his answers to the 15 questions identified seven major themes. These included, tension, knowledge, professional competence and several themes relating to cultural aspects of the workplace, for example the low value placed on learning. His self-confidence declined from moderate to low during the first two months of his employment and, by the end of the fifth month, it had reached a moderate level again.

In an attempt to generalize her findings, Boyd Boonyauiroj takes trouble to relate them to other studies of physiotherapists returning to work and to theories relating to role transition and professional socialization. She states:

> Although some of Martin's recorded experiences and reactions would be peculiar to him and his reason for absence, others would be pertinent to returning physiotherapists of all grades who have taken time out for different reasons and purposes, such as child rearing. (1996: 447)

Her research subject, a male physiotherapist who had taken a career break to obtain a PhD is, however, atypical of most physiotherapists which makes it more difficult to generalize the findings. However, some of his experiences, for example low self-confidence and a poor learning environment, are likely to generalize. Kvale states that generalization in qualitative research

> ... involves a reasoned judgement about the extent to which the findings of one study can be used as a guide to what might occur in another situation. It is based on an analysis of the similarities and differences of the two situations ... By specifying the supporting arguments and making the arguments explicit, the researcher can allow readers to judge the soundness of the generalization claim. (Kvale 1996: 233)

The choice of the particular case always needs to be justified. When deciding among equally suitable alternatives pragmatic decisions based upon convenience are legitimate.

Smith and Topping (1996) undertook a case study with three physically disabled children to see how well they could use a robotic aid for drawing. The children were observed undertaking various drawing tasks and then one child was observed intensively to discover how well he could do what the other children in the class were doing. The child and the classroom teacher were also given questionnaires to complete on the usefulness of the robotic aid and the enjoyment and satisfaction it gave as well as their suggestions for improvement in the design.

Tryssenaar (1999) conducted a case study to investigate the lived experience of the first four months of practice of an occupational therapist. Two interviews were conducted as well as written answers to open-ended questions. The data obtained indicated an initial period of enthusiasm and optimism which rapidly gave way to lack of confidence, disappointment and dissatisfaction with working within an atmosphere of low morale, strikes and confusing inter-professional boundaries. Finally the occupational therapist took measures to protect herself such as avoiding people who were dissatisfied and actively seeking support.

> **Stop and Think**
> What value do you think a case study of this type may have?
> Write down the ways in which the information from this
> case study could be used to benefit other occupational
> therapists.

You may consider this to be an isolated case that cannot be generalized. The findings do, however, tally with larger studies of professional socialization which show a similar pattern. It also gives a lot of very detailed information that would be lost with many research methods such as a large survey. Tryssenaar believes that this case study indicates a need for educational changes for occupational therapy students and support for newly qualified occupational therapists. She states:

> Understanding the lived experience of becoming an occupational therapist has implications for educational programmes. These could incorporate the inclusion and expansion of organizational politics into the curriculum and provide formal recognition and support for mentoring of new graduates by supervisors, experienced clinicians and academics. (1999: 111)

The opportunity to use several methods (a multi-method approach) is a further advantage of the case study approach. The use of multiple sources of evidence strengthens the validity of the data and allows a more holistic interpretation. It is more likely than a single method to capture the depth and complexity of a situation. Yin states:

> No matter how the experience is gained, every case study investigator should be well versed in a variety of data collection techniques so that a case study can use multiple sources of evidence. Without such multiple sources, an invaluable advantage of the case study strategy will have been lost. (1994: 94)

The case study approach may help to make the research process more democratic. In some ways it may be easier for 'non-researchers' or novice researchers to take part in case studies than in large scale research projects because they do not need to secure large amounts of funding and may be able to undertake the research as part of their everyday work. This is not to imply that case study research is easy; Yin (1984) points out that it is difficult to make use of research assistants in case study research because the studies depend on the ability to link theoretical issues to the data being collected in order to take advantage of unexpected opportunities and to interpret the research findings. Researchers must, therefore, be adaptable and flexible with a sound grasp of the theoretical issues in question. As noted above, they should also have knowledge of a range of research methods.

The results of case studies tend to be more comprehensive, intelligible and interesting to many people than more traditional research reports, which are sometimes full of statistical tables, complicated graphs and jargon. Thus the case study approach assists in the dissemination of knowledge, helping to make it accessible to a wider readership. However, a shortcoming of case study research is that insufficient effort tends to be given to the formation of a comprehensive database which can be retrieved and scrutinized by interested persons. Such a database could include the researcher's notes, interview transcripts and observation schedules.

Limitations of the case study approach

> **Stop and Think**
> Having read about the advantages of case study research, what do you consider the disadvantages to be? Write a list of the possible disadvantages using your own experience if appropriate.

It is often said that case studies are suitable to explore or describe a situation but not to explain it; there are certainly many uncontrolled variables which render causal explanations difficult to make. Yin, however, disagrees. He believes that information from case studies can be used to '... explain the causal links in real-life interventions that are too complex for the surveyor experimental strategies'. (1994: 15) Thus case studies can be used for testing theory as well as building theory (Denscombe, 1998). Researchers need, however, to avoid 'selective bias' whereby they select only those parts of the data that support their theories.

Another frequently mentioned limitation of case studies is that the resulting data is specific to the particular case and therefore cannot be generalized to others. However, although the logic of the case study is to gain specific insights, these insights usually have wider implications, as Arksey and Knight state '... the general is always present in the particular'. (1999: 58) Generalization is possible if the case is chosen because it is 'typical', conversely if extreme cases provide evidence to support an underlying theory then the theory has greater validity. Generalization also becomes possible if case studies are replicated. A number of therapists may, for example, be undertaking case studies of patients with a particular medical condition which, together, will build up a body of theory. 'Limitations', such as the inability to generalize, are always relative to the particular approach being taken in research.

A further difficulty with case studies is knowing precisely what 'the case' is. This is relatively easy if it is an individual but more difficult if it is a ward, a department or a hospital. The boundaries of the case need to be thought through carefully before the research commences.

Conclusion

The case study, particularly when focusing on a single person, is a very manageable research approach for practising therapists. It gives an opportunity to use a variety of methods and to study a particular situation in depth. If the aim is to assist a particular patient or client then an inability to generalize will not be important, but case studies frequently give important insights which can be used far beyond the particular case.

Analysing data

Starting points: What have you found?

That recurring question, 'And what have you found so far?' can be the most threatening and anxiety-provoking of all to researchers. As we shall see in Part One of this chapter, questions of the analysis of quantitative data centre mainly around patterns in the social and physical world, revealed through the use of numbers and statistics. In Part Two, we turn to the analysis of qualitative data and the many and varied stories and meanings of personal experiences in the social world.

Part one: Analysing quantitative data

There is much you can do with quantitative data with only basic arithmetic and the use of graphs. If in addition you approach quantitative analysis on a gradual 'need to know' basis, and are willing to practise with increasingly available statistical software packages (such as SPSS), you will gradually master more advanced forms of analysis.

Quantitative data may be analysed using descriptive or inferential approaches. Descriptive statistics basically summarize the data, helping you to determine patterns that cannot be seen 'by eye' in your data such as differences between groups, or associations between two variables. Inferential statistics encompass many tests which help you to determine whether the patterns in your data conform to your hypothesis – for example, whether the differences in scores in two groups are really likely to have occurred only by chance or whether they possibly reflect a genuine experimental (or treatment) effect. An understanding of statistical significance is required when interpreting inferential statistics. Before proceeding further, it is important for you to appreciate the type of data that your project is collecting. Your choice of descriptive or inferential statistic will depend on you getting this right!

Levels of measurement

Although all your research data may exist in the form of numbers, there may be a different logic underlying each measurement. It is important that you understand the level of measurement in order to determine the appropriate statistic. Take the following hypothetical example:

A researcher is studying the effects of a back pain management programme. The measures taken from all participants included the following:

- Attendance (measured as either 'completion of programme' = 1/'drop-out' = 0).
- Pain rating on a 0–10 scale (where 0 = no pain at all and 10 = worst possible pain).
- Time taken to walk a set distance, in seconds.

The scores collected reflect a nominal, ordinal and ratio level of measurement respectively.

The nominal level of measurement
With this scale, the numbers classify the data into categories. Each number acts as a label rather than signifying a quantity. In the above example, 'drop-outs' could have been classed as 'I' and 'attenders' as '0'. Sex and marital status may also be 'nominal'. It does not make sense to carry out certain mathematical operations on these scores – for example to say that

Table 15.1 Hypothetical set of data taken at the end of a 6-week pain management programme

Participant	Attendance	Pain Rating (0–10)	Time for Walk (sec)
1.	1	7	62
2.	1	6	55
3.	1	8	75
4.	0	8	78
5.	1	4	50
6.	0	6	58

average attendance score was 4/6 (0.67) as the codes (1 or 0) are arbitrary and the resulting figure applies to no-one in the sample. Instead, you should report on the number of the sample being classified into each category (e.g. there were 4 attenders and 2 non-attenders).

The ordinal level of measurement
Here, the data can be ranked or ordered in terms of size. From Table 15.1, Participant 3 is clearly reporting greater pain (rating of 8) than Participant 5 (rating of 4). Likert scales (see Chapter 8) are also ordinal in nature. Although we can determine which are larger or smaller scores, the numbers are not necessarily spread equally along the scale. Participant 5 reports less pain, yet we cannot be sure it is genuinely 'half' the pain of Participant 3.

There is much debate about the appropriate way of analysing ordinal data. Because the intervals between the points on the scale may vary in size, some argue that one should not add, divide, multiply or subtract ordinal data. Instead of calculating a mean, other forms of averaging may be used (see later). Choice of inferential test is also affected. Despite these arguments, ordinal scores are added together to achieve an overall total on many standardized scales (such as the Hospital Anxiety and Depression Scale – HADS). It is recommended that you seek statistical advice if you consider treating your own ordinal data in this way.

The interval scale

On interval scales, there is an equal distance between each point on the scale. Most 'public' or objective measuring tools such as tape measures, weighing scales and clocks provide interval data. The time to walk a set distance (in the example above) provides an example of interval data.

Because the scale points are equally spaced, it makes sense to add and subtract scores. From Table 15.1, we can calculate that Participant 2 is 20 seconds faster than Participant 3. Participant 5 takes two thirds of the time that Participant 3 required. There is a particular type of interval scale called the *ratio* scale, which has a meaningful zero. Time, weight, length, angles and so on are measured on ratio scales. However, some interval scales have essentially a 'man-made' or artificial zero. One example is temperature measured on the Celsius scale, because zero is arbitrarily defined as the freezing point of water (not alcohol, nitrogen or any other substance!).

Descriptive statistics

It is often impossible to detect patterns or make comparisons by viewing a large matrix of numbers. Both descriptive statistics and graphical methods of presentation both provide ways of making quantitative data manageable and easier to comprehend. The most common descriptive summaries are measures of central tendency (averages) and measures of the dispersion (or spread) of the scores.

Measures of central tendency

There are three types of average, namely the mean, median and mode. They have different uses and choice is shaped by whether the data are ordinal or interval.

Mean

This is found by adding scores together and then dividing the total by the number of scores in the list. In Table 15.1, the walking times of 6 participants are given. To work out the mean, add the six 'walking times' (making 378) and divide by the number of participants (6). The mean is 63 seconds. If you also had the data taken before the intervention programme began, you could tell whether the average time had decreased (or not) – that is, whether patients were becoming (on average) more mobile after treatment.

The mean is less useful when there are unusually extreme (or 'outlying') scores within the data-set. Imagine that a 7th patient's walking speed is very slow (180 seconds). If we take the mean of the seven scores (the six in Table 15.1 and the seventh one of 180 seconds), the mean increases to 79.7 seconds. This number is not representative of the original six patients, and so an alternative form of average might be less misleading, such as the median.

Median
If you place your scores in order of size and find the *middle* score, you have the median. For example, 50, 55, 58, 62, 75, 78 reflects the rank ordering of the 'walking time' scores. There is an even number of scores (6) so the median is found by adding the two middle scores together (58 + 62) and finding their mean (i.e. 58 + 62 = 120; divided by 2). The median is therefore 60.

The median is less affected by extreme scores than the mean. For example, if we add the very slow time of 180 to the original set of six, the median only changes from 60 to 62 (50, 55, 58, 62, 75, 78, 180). The median may be an appropriate average when the data are ordinal, as it is questionable to add or divide scores that are not drawn from an interval scale.

Stop and Think
Find the median of the Pain Ratings in Table 15.1.

(Answer is at the end of the chapter).

Mode
The mode is the most frequently occurring score within a data set, and thereby describes the most typical measurement. It is

most useful for describing nominal data. For example, looking at the 'attendance' figures in Table 15.1, the mode is 1 (the code representing attendance). The mode indicates that most patients (4/6) attended the programme.

Although modal scores can also be determined for ordinal and interval data, if every score is different (e.g. 'Walk Times'), there is no 'modal' value. There can also be several modes in a set of numbers, (look at the pain ratings in Table 15.1), rendering this measure less useful, especially for small sets of data.

Measures of variability
Measures of variability express the amount of spread or dispersion in the scores. There are several measures, with range and standard deviation widely used. The range is the simplest measure of 'spread' of scores. It is calculated by subtracting the lowest score in a set of numbers from the highest score. Returning to the Pain Ratings data (Table 15.1), the range is 4, as the highest score is 8 and the lowest is 4 (8 − 4 = 4). Whilst the range is simple to calculate, it is very much affected by extreme scores. Particularly with interval data, variance or standard deviation may be preferred. We approach our first formula! But beforehand, let us try to understand what 'variance' means. We will take another hypothetical set of data to illustrate.

Example: A specialist team audit the number of home visits that they carry out each month for one year. They compare the number of visits carried out monthly in the 'winter' half of the year, and in the 'summer' half. The data are shown in Table 15.2.

Stop and Think
Check why the mean does not offer a complete, fair summary of the pattern of visits in each half-year.

Despite the same mean number of visits, you will have noticed (hopefully) that the range of scores in the winter months is much more variable than in the summer months. Indeed, the range for the winter half-year is 14 (28 − 14) and the range for the summer

Table 15.2 Audit Data for Home Visits (Hypothetical)

Winter half-year		Summer half-year	
Month	No. Home visits	Month	No. Home visits
September	20	March	22
October	16	April	20
November	18	May	18
December	14	June	16
January	24	July	22
February	28	August	22
Mean no. visits/month (Winter)	20	Mean no. visits/month (Summer)	20

half-year is 6 (22 − 16). Another way of showing the variation in scores is provided by calculating how far each score differs from the mean (which was 20 visits on average per month as shown in Table 15.2), and then calculating the *variance*. We will do this for the winter half-year data (see Table 15.3).

As the scores are spread above and below the mean, the positive and negative differences add to zero (column 3). Whilst the difference scores (deviations from the mean) provide an indication of 'spread', they cannot be simply added together as the negatives and positives cancel each other out. As often happens in statistical calculations, to overcome this the difference scores are squared (each score is multiplied by itself), as can be seen in the last column. When negative numbers are squared they become positive, so this removes the problem of minus numbers. The deviations (squared) are added together (Σ, pronounced 'sigma', stands for 'sum of'). In this case the total = 136 (column 4). This

Table 15.3 First step in calculating the variance in the number of monthly visits in the 'winter' half-year data

Month	No. visits/month	Difference between the monthly figure and mean (20)	Difference^2
Sept	20	(20 – 20) = 0	0
Oct	16	(16 – 20) = –4	16
Nov	18	(18 – 20) = –2	4
Dec	14	(14 – 20) = –6	36
Jan	24	(24 – 20) = +4	16
Feb	28	(28 – 20) = +8	64

^{2}Sum of (Σ) differences = 136

total is then divided by the sample size (6 scores, relating to 6 months' figures) to establish the mean squared deviation – or *variance*.

The mean squared deviation is 136/6 = 22.67

To summarize, this procedure is set out by the formula:

$$\text{Variance} = \frac{\Sigma\,(S - M)^2}{N}$$

(where S = score; M = mean of scores; N = number of scores; Σ = sum of)

This formula estimates the variance in the sample itself. To estimate the variance in the population more generally, the formula is adapted slightly to:

$$\text{Variance} = \frac{\Sigma\,(S - M)^2}{N - 1}$$

Standard deviation
The standard deviation (SD) is derived from the square root of the variance (in other words, the SD multiplied by itself equals the variance). In the above case, the square root of 22.67 = 4.8.

209

Many research results are reported in terms of standard deviation rather than variance, possibly because the measure, being in the same units of measurement as the original data, can be more directly compared with the individual scores and the mean.

The larger the SD the greater the spread of a given set of scores around the mean. With a normal distribution of scores, approximately 68% of the data are found within 1 standard deviation above and below the mean, and 95% of scores occur within 2 SDs. Scores found beyond this realm are unusual and may indicate the need for some attention. For example, a child who is more than two SDs underweight for their age may require urgent nutritional intervention.

Stop and Think
1. Calculate the SD for the summer half-year data, and compare the value to the winter SD (of 4.8) shown above.
2. Taking the twelve months of data as a whole, find the mode and median scores. The mean is already known (20).

Inferential statistics

Once you have explored your data in a descriptive way, you may wish to determine whether the results from your sample can really be generalized to the wider population. You may be seeking to establish whether groups 'really' or 'significantly' differ in their responses, for example, before and after treatment. Inferential statistics help you to do this. Simple statistical tests usually examine *differences* between two sets of scores or *associations* (correlations) between variables. More complex tests can examine the combined effects of more than one variable at a time.

Statistical significance
In establishing whether results are statistically significant or not, we are essentially selecting between competing hypotheses, a

null hypothesis and an alternative (research) hypothesis. In the pain/mobility example already given, the researcher can test the following hypotheses:

- Null hypothesis: there is no relationship between pain ratings and walking times.
- Alternative hypothesis: there is a positive correlation between pain ratings and walking times.

This alternative hypothesis is known as 'one-tailed' or 'directional' because it specifies the direction of association. Directional hypotheses are usually adopted when there is sufficient previous evidence to support a firm prediction. Exploratory (or 'two-tailed') hypotheses do not specify direction. For example, the researcher may simply predict a difference between two groups without stating which group will score higher, or may predict a correlation without specifying whether it is positive or negative. Exploratory hypotheses are more common in new fields of enquiry about which little is known.

The statistical test allows us to accept or reject the null hypothesis, with a probability known as the significance level. If the test is 'significant', then the pattern of data is sufficiently extreme for the null hypothesis to be considered unlikely. By default, the research (or alternative) hypothesis – that there is a genuine effect – is then accepted. However, it can never be 'proven'.

Significance levels are expressed in terms of probability (e.g. $p = 0.05$). When we conclude that results (differences or correlations) are significant at the 0.05 level, we are saying that there is 0.05 (or 5%) probability of rejecting the null hypothesis when it is true. It essentially represents the probability of making a mistake, believing there to be a 'genuine' effect where there is none. This is called the 'Type 1' error. If a therapist compares two groups of patients following different treatments and finds that their outcome measures are different at the 0.05 level of significance, the inference is drawn that there is a genuine effect of treatment – one is more effective than the other. Nevertheless, the 0.05 (or 5%) refers to the probability that this result may have occurred without there being any genuine differences between the groups – the null hypothesis still has a low (5%) chance of being 'true'. The lower the probability level (e.g. 0.01 or 0.001) the less risk there is of rejecting the null hypothesis falsely. However, if results are accepted as significant *only* when the probability of a Type 1 error is very low (requiring p < 0.01, say), then the 'Type 2' error becomes more likely – accepting the null hypothesis when it is in fact wrong.

This reasoning shows why the errors are sometimes referred to as: Type 1 error – optimistic (rejecting the null hypothesis when correct – optimistically accepting that there is an 'experimental' effect); Type 2 error – pessimistic (accepting the null hypothesis when incorrect – being too cautious about accepting our experimental effects).

Statistical significance should not be equated with clinical significance. With very large samples, it is quite easy for even small differences or associations within the data to be statistically significant, but they may not have any clinical implications. Equally, a result which is 'non-significant' is not uninteresting or a 'failure' or clinically irrelevant. There can be many reasons for not obtaining the patterns that we expect in our data. Poor research design and insufficient sample size can of course be responsible but it is also possible that our basic theory needs re-examining. A non-significant result can indicate that previous evidence (or clinical 'accepted wisdom') is not as strong as we believed it to be, and it may generate many hypotheses to guide further research. Non-significant differences between treatment groups can also be very important for establishing that a more expensive intervention is not cost-effective.

Choosing an appropriate statistical test
Many books provide a 'decision tree' to aid the choice of which statistical test to select (e.g. Greene & D'Oliveira, 1999). Assuming you have chosen a simple research design, you basically need to ask:

● Am I analysing differences or associations between scores?
● Do I have a related design or an independent groups design?
● Are my data measured at the nominal, ordinal or interval levels?

- Are my data reasonably normally distributed, or seriously skewed?
- Do my two sets of scores show fairly similar standard deviations?

If the data are ordinal, and particularly if they show skewed distributions, and/or very different standard deviations, the usual advice is to choose a *non-parametric* test (which sets out fewer requirements about the data), whereas normally distributed interval data may be processed using *parametric* tests. It is often 'safer' to select non-parametric tests as they can process a wider variety of data types, but they are less powerful – in other words, they are less likely to be able to reject the null hypothesis. The reader is recommended to Coolidge (2000), Diamantopoulos & Schlegelmich (1997) or Greene & D'Oliveira (1999) to find out more details about choosing an inferential test.

Part two: Analysing qualitative data

One way of looking at the analysis of qualitative data is the building of a story which encapsulates and expresses the main themes arising from the data collected, though it is never the only possible story. Analysis is a process of bringing order to those 'piles' of data, organizing the data and searching for patterns. Analysing also involves interpretation, offering explanations for the emerging patterns and attaching meaning to the emerging themes. Huberman and Miles (1994) provide a useful breakdown of the process of analysis:

- *Data reduction:* This refers to the process of selecting, focusing, simplifying, abstracting and transforming 'raw data'.
- *Data display:* This refers to the organized assembly of information that permits conclusion drawing and action taking.
- *Drawing conclusions/verification:* This refers to the process of deciding what things mean, including noting regularities, patterns, explanations, possible configurations, causal flows and propositions.

Analysis, including interpretation, is the crucial foundation for clarity, rigour and a systematic approach to qualitative research. Analysis is, however, also a creative and challenging process requiring continual reflection. It is not usually a distinct stage or phase of research. It begins at the planning stage, shapes the formulation and use of data collection methods, and continues into the process of writing up. Indeed, in some qualitative research data analysis and collection build on each other. Thus, data are collected, analysed, and then further data are collected on the basis of the analysis.

Some research projects involve the collection of both qualitative and quantitative data, for example where a questionnaire is used to collect information from clients about, say, how often they experience breathlessness, the time of the day they experience breathlessness, and unstructured interviews are conducted with a few clients to explore their experiences in detail. There are advantages to this. A major advantage of open-ended questions is that they put 'flesh on the bones' of statistical data, and research is usually strengthened if more than one mode of analysis is used.

Emerging themes

There are a variety of ways of approaching the analysis of qualitative research. A commonly used approach, and a useful approach for beginner researchers, is *content analysis*. As Denscombe states:

> ... it is a method that can be used with any 'text' whether it be in the form of writings, sounds or pictures, as a way of quantifying the content of that text. (1998: 167–168)

This type of analysis is a search for the patterns and categories that emerge, or recur, within the data. The process is one of looking for quotations or observations which go together as examples or expressions of the same underlying idea, issue or concept. It is, or should be, a search for differences as much as a search for consensus. It is an extremely time-consuming aspect of the research, consisting of hours of 'listen-

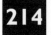

ing' to the data, reading and re-reading transcripts, field notes and documents.

The starting point is the data, and this will depend on the method of data collection.

Open-ended and semi-structured interviews
If the interviews were tape-recorded the researcher should transcribe them from the tape into a verbatim script. This process is very time-consuming. A common question from students is, 'do I have to transcribe the interviews?' We would strongly recommend that you do as transcription is the best starting point for analysis. If you do not transcribe interviews fully, then you should listen repeatedly to the tapes to pick out recurring themes and make a note of significant quotations.

Open-ended questions in questionnaires
Analysing open questions is generally more time-consuming than analysing closed questions. Although research participants may express their ideas in many different ways, they may be covering just a few basic ideas.

Unstructured observation
The data is likely to be in the form of hand-written notes. These notes may include descriptions of events, theoretical analyses, details of methods and the researcher's own feelings and perceptions. If possible, events observed should be recorded immediately to minimize errors and distortions of memory.

Documents
When undertaking a content analysis, it is necessary to formulate the research question, and then to define and select the documents to be analysed.

The following are the basic steps of content analysis.

1. Read and analyse
The data should be read and an analysis undertaken that summarizes and thus reduces, but also accurately reflects the substance of the data. Let us assume, for instance, that you are interested in the ways in which disabled people are presented in

the popular press and have decided to analyse a random sample of magazine articles on disability and disabled people. The first step is to read the articles through and jot down all the ways in which disabled people are described. For example they may be described as pitiful, heroic, asexual, superhuman or 'normal'. In analysing an interview transcript you are similarly attempting to reduce the data to the key ideas being expressed without distorting them. This can be quite difficult as all data has a manifest and a latent content. Manifest content refers to the visible, surface content of data, whereas latent content refers to its underlying meaning. Manifest content is more objective but latent content is often more revealing. Whether researchers concentrate on the manifest or the latent content of the data, depends on their underlying research questions. Concentrating on latent content involves 'reading between the lines' and taking note of what is not said. This is most valuable if it can be backed up with other evidence. As you undertake the first step, you need to make notes on recurring themes in the data. In the above example this would involve deciding whether any of the descriptions are so similar that they can be combined into one category.

2. List themes/categories

Draw up a list of the main recurring themes/categories. Write a short definition of each theme. Returning to the above example, this would involve devising a simple chart (category frame) within which to record the various descriptions of disability. The categories must be exhaustive which means that it should be possible to categorize every relevant item, and mutually exclusive, which means that no item can be recorded in more than one category. It is permissible to have an 'other' category but this should be avoided if possible. It can be helpful, and may improve reliability, if several people assist with the task of devising categories. Deciding on the categories to be used can be problematic; too few may limit the data, reducing its validity, but too many may make categorization difficult and reliability poor. Researchers are advised to undertake this work as quickly as possible after the interviews while the information is still fresh in their minds. A content analysis is no better than its categories.

Reliability is greatest when categories are clearly stated and do not overlap. Fine discriminations may be difficult to code but may be extremely important.

3. Re-analyse and re-categorize
You are now in a position to look again at the data very carefully to analyse their content using the category frame. You may also write down any quotations that add substance to the data and any ideas and perceptions which may assist with your interpretation and presentation of the results. During this step, the framework of categories might change, with definitions of categories being clarified and, sometimes, new categories emerging as you look again. It is important to make a note of data, such as things people say in the interviews, that either seem to fit into more than one category or not into any. These data can help in clarifying categories and in seeing the relationships between categories.

Stop and Think
Select a short article from a magazine such as *Therapy Weekly* and undertake a content analysis to find the major themes within the article. Select any quotations which illustrate your themes.

Variations on a theme

While a version of content analysis can be a good starting point for therapists new to qualitative research, it may also be useful to look at some different approaches. This is not easy as it was possible to distinguish among twenty-six different kinds of approach to qualitative research over ten years ago (Tesch, 1990). It is possible, however, to group the kinds of approaches.

Coding and categorizing

These approaches aim to reduce the data by paraphrasing, summarizing and categorizing (Flick, 1998). Content analysis is one such approach. Another comprehensive approach is 'theoretical coding' which is part of a research process aimed at developing 'grounded theories', that is theories which arise from the analysis and interpretation of data (Strauss and Corbin, 1998).

Holistic and sequential

There are a number of approaches to analysis which focus on 'the ways in which social actors produce, represent, and contextualize experience and personal knowledge through narratives and other genres' (Coffey and Atkinson, 1996: 54). Though these approaches differ in important ways, they tend to: focus on the views, or stories, of each participant, rather than searching for recurring themes across participants; interpret what participants say or do as part of a sequence of interaction, rather than taking quotations, or any data, out of the immediate context; and interpretations also take account of the broader social and historic context.

Narrative analyses, for instance, require the researcher to develop a reflective stance in considering what factors influenced the flow of the conversation between the interviewer and participant. Kohler Riessman suggests that analysis of a narrative interview should begin with the interviewer asking herself the following questions about the structure of the narrative. 'How is (the narrative) organized? Why does the informant develop her tale this way in conversation with this listener?' She goes on to say that these strategies, together with identifying underlying propositions – what is taken for granted by the listener and the teller – give greater weight to the participant's experience (1993: 61).

Narrative analysis of interviews requires researchers to interpret and deconstruct the experience of the narrator in terms of structural and institutional factors that influence identity and shape the experience. As Goodley suggests:

We hear the personal reminiscences of the storyteller and at the same time, are drawn to the broader, structural horizons which function as a backdrop to the narrative. (1996: 337)

Computer-assisted analysis

Many approaches can be supported by the use of computer packages. We do not think that computer-assisted analysis is an approach in its own right. Like Coffey and Atkinson (1998), we believe that it is important to identify your strategy for analysis before turning to the computer for all the practical assistance it can offer. Various computer packages, for example NUDIST and ETHNOGRAPH, have been devised to assist with the analysis of qualitative data. Though these can be useful, a good word processing package such as Word for Windows will be sufficient for the needs of most beginner researchers.

Conclusion

Those of you who are quite new to research should feel reassured that much can be gleaned from your data using descriptive analysis and graphical representations. Inferential tests provide further useful tools for testing research hypotheses, and can be explored on a 'need-to-know' basis. However it is approached, a qualitative analysis is essentially about quality in the social world and people's lives and experiences: similarities and differences, subtleties and nuances, variety and change; themes, sub-themes and variations on themes.

Answers to 'Stop & Think' Exercises 1, 2 & 3

Exercise 1: The median is found between the middle figures 6 and 7.

Exercise 2: The middle scorers (position 30–31 out of 60) fall between depression scores 11–15. This is also the modal category (most frequently occurring).

Exercise 3: (a) The sample variance is 5.3, and the SD is 2.3. (b) The modal number of visits is 22 (as there are 3 months in which 22 visits took place). The median number is 20, taken from the middle scores of the ranked data – 14, 16, 16, 18, 18, 20, 20, 22, 22, 22, 24, 28.

Narrative approaches to research

with Maureen Gillman

Introduction: Sitting comfortably?

Over the past two decades narrative methods of research have increased in popularity and have become a significant part of the repertoire of researchers from a wide range of disciplines, including psychology, social work, psychotherapy, education – and therapy. Narrative approaches to researching include life history, life story, oral history and autobiography. Hollway and Jefferson characterize narrative approaches as those in which 'the researcher's responsibility is to be a good listener and the interviewee is a story-teller rather than a respondent … the agenda is open to development and change, depending on the narrator's experiences' (2000: 31). These methods of narrative research share a common perception that people live their lives by stories, and that such stories are not just accounts of peoples' lives but they are also shaping and constitutive of their identities. Writing of the link between identity and narrative life history, Widdershoven states: 'What then is narrative identity? It is the unity of a person's life as it is experienced and articulated in stories that express this experience … the unity of a person's life is dependent on being a character in an enacted narrative. We live our lives according to a script, which secures that our actions are part of a meaningful totality. Our actions are organized in such a way that we can give account of them, justify them by telling an intelligible story about them' (1993: 7). Narrative research methods can give voice to the experience of people, particularly oppressed groups, by celebrating their strengths and challenging negative stereotypes.

What is narrative research?

The focus of inquiry for the narrative researcher is the 'story', that is, first person accounts by respondents of their experience, whilst the purpose of narrative analysis is:

> ... to see how respondents in interviews impose order on the flow of experience to make sense of events and actions in their lives. The question is, 'Why was the story told that way?' (Kohler Reissman, 1993: 2).

Narrative research methods fall within an interpretivist framework of research, which is the study, expression and interpretation of subjective human experience. Whilst positivism seeks to discover facts and causal relationships, and to generate formal, sometimes grand theories, interpretivism asks how lived experience and interaction is organized, perceived and constructed. Whilst positivists seek to separate themselves from the world they study, interpretivists choose to participate in that world, and see the research process itself as a legitimate subject for inquiry. Some key assumptions about the interpretivist paradigm are:

- For any situation a potentially unlimited number of descriptions and explanations is possible.
- Reality derives from human interaction aimed at 'meaning making'.
- Such meaning exists only through social agreement and consensus amongst participants.
- Reality is constructed within a context and can change as the context changes.
- Research is value laden.

Whilst positivist researchers would be concerned about the facts, accuracy and truth status of a participant's story, the narrative researcher makes no such distinction and argues that human agency and imagination determine what is included and what is left out of the story. Kohler Reissman suggests that,

> A personal narrative is not meant to be read as an exact record of what happened, nor is it a mirror of a world 'out there' ... Telling about complex and troubling events should vary because the past is a selective reconstruction. (1993: 64)

Widdershoven argues that life is a story put into practice. In order to make sense of life, people need to have access to the 'stock of stories that constitute its dramatic resources' (1993: 4). Life histories and stories are not just a description of a series of factual events, but narratives that are shaped and structured in the telling of the story.

There are moments or experiences in a person's life that change or leave marks on the individual. Denzin (1989) describes such events as 'personal epiphanies'. Many clients in occupational therapy and physiotherapy have experienced or are experiencing 'personal epiphanies'. This can include clients with head injuries, neurological disorders and elderly people, especially those with stroke or dementing illness. An example of a 'personal epiphany' in my own life (M.G.), its meaning and the power of the story to shape identity and life events, may help to clarify the above. When I was ten years old, I went with my mother to see a consultant ophthalmologist at a local hospital. After examination he told my mother, in my presence, that my sight was very poor and likely to deteriorate further. His advice to my mother was that I would never amount to much and should be guided away from employment in which I would need to read and write. He thought some kind of practical work with my hands would be a suitable direction for me. My mother was incensed by this advice and, with a rather rude comment to the consultant, we left. I can remember her indignation and her subsequent determination to refute this predicted future for me and I recall a growing determination, on my part, to prove him wrong. The consultant's predictions about my sight proved to be accurate and I am now registered blind. However, his prophecy about my abilities and subsequent employment have not materialized. I stayed in mainstream education and eventually trained as a social worker. Since then I have obtained a PhD and I am employed as a Principal Lecturer at a University.

I use this story in my teaching on disability studies in the university, as a way of demonstrating the power of the medical model of disability to shape identities and to exclude disabled people from mainstream society. However, it is also a story I use to make sense of the direction of my own life and my achievements.

Stop and Think

Identify a 'personal epiphany' in your own life and write it down. Reflect upon the images and feelings it provokes. How has the meaning you have constructed from this event shaped your subsequent experiences and life events?

A study by McKay and Ryan (1995) is an example of a narrative approach in therapy research. It is based on the idea that narrative reasoning is a means of enabling occupational therapists to explain their practice. A student and an experienced therapist were asked to tell their story about one particular client with whom they were working. The experienced therapist 'presented a future or conditional image of the person which guided the intervention: "it's up to us to get her home"' (p 236). The student's story, however, kept strictly to the formal therapy process.

Forms of narrative research

There are a number of different methods which come under the umbrella of narrative research. We shall look in more detail at just two: oral history, the review of history through personal reminiscence; and life history, an account of a person's life that includes biographical information. The latter can include: autobiography, where the person is the sole author of the story; and life story, an account of an event or events in a person's life.

Oral history

Atkinson suggests that oral history involves people remembering past personal and social events and:

> ... often includes people who have been neglected in traditional history books, such as working class people, women and mental health survivors. (1993b: 59)

In documenting the experiences of 'ordinary people', oral historians represent a challenge to traditional forms of historical accounts which are based on documentary 'evidence'. Bornat argues that accounts of the lived experience of ordinary people challenges historical and political orthodoxies (1993: 85). Oral sources can provide a basis for the re-examination of well-documented spheres through new perspectives. For example Okihiro argues that outsiders rather than the people themselves have written ethnic history. It is a 'colonized' history, an apt metaphor when considering the history of people whose land was colonized. He states:

> Oral history proposes that we rewrite our history to capture the human spirit of the people to see how ethnic minorities solved or failed to solve particular problems, how they advanced or resisted change, and how they made or failed to make better lives for themselves and their children. In short, oral history proposes nothing less than the writing of a people's history, liberated from myths and imbued with humanity. (1981: 211)

Oral historians have a particularly important role in bringing forth the marginalized and subjugated voices of people with learning difficulties. Their exclusion from mainstream society in the form of institutionalization has meant that the history of people with learning difficulties in our society has been colonized and written by others. Atkinson describes how the participants in an oral history group came to an awareness that past ideas such as policies and labels, impinged upon and changed their lives. She goes on to say that:

In the telling and retelling of her story, Mabel has demonstrated how important it is for people with learning difficulties to have and to own a history which is theirs. (1999: 20)

Whilst oral history research has an important role in challenging dominant discourses about people with learning difficulties (and other marginalized groups), the telling and reclaiming of personal history also has other, perhaps less obvious benefits for the participants. Atkinson asserts that:

Being an oral historian and a contributor to a written history have brought other, less tangible rewards to the people concerned. Their new roles have increased self-confidence and an enhanced sense of self ... to have that past put into a written format which can be shown and shared is to gain recognition as a person who matters. (1993b: v)

Atkinson also suggests that:

The challenge is for people, including therapists, who work with those with learning difficulties to play their part in the telling of more stories. Therapists are well placed through their work and in their relationships with people with learning difficulties to play an active part in the telling of stories. This starts with recognizing that everyone has a personal past, and acknowledging and respecting that past. (1999: 21)

Life history

There is no clearly defined delineation between oral and life history, as there is no absolute distinction between 'social' and 'personal' histories. Social history is embedded in personal histories, just as a personal history is embedded in social history. Oral and life history are narrative methods: the telling of personal and social histories.

Life histories are not just a series of factual events, but narratives that are shaped and structured in the telling of the story. Individuals tell stories about their lives in order to make sense of their lives. Stories are therefore important for identity as they tell us who we are. Lack or loss of personal history has an effect on the stories people tell about themselves. People can lose personal histories in many different circumstances including institutionalization and the development of dementia or memory loss following brain injury. In the absence of information, it is possible that the person concerned will adopt a fatalistic attitude to life, or use fantasy to fill in the gaps (Heyman *et al*, 1997). Professionals may also use such strategies to fill in the information gaps of those in their care. The difference is that their speculations are regarded as having a higher 'truth' status as they are often supported by theoretical discourse. (Gillman *et al*, 1997). McCarthy (1994) makes the point that information about the ordinary life of an individual is confirming sameness rather than accentuating difference, whereas information constructed through professional discourse has a tendency to be 'problem saturated' and pathologizing. The stories that we tell ourselves and others about our histories are influential in constructing identities and making connections between ourselves and others. An absence of personal history leaves individuals open to having a history and a subsequent identity imposed upon them by others more powerful than themselves. The telling of personal history can be significant for the listener as well as the narrator. The life histories of frail elderly people, for instance, may speak to the powerful roles that clients had taken in their younger days. They can help therapists challenge the infantilizing of the person in daily care practices.

The major strengths of life history research is in its attendance to the insider view and the depiction of experience in ways that are faithful to the meaning given by the persons concerned. It has the potential to challenge hitherto 'unquestionable truths' and 'remind us of the lives behind the label' (Goodley, 1996: 333). Life history research also allows for the exploration of areas of life that written records scarcely touch. In recent research we found that many respondents looked to the written records of professionals to provide background information and personal history material but they frequently found that the kind of information they were seeking was not contained in the 'official' records. Yet such records are often inaccessible (both literally and conceptually) to those who are the subjects of their deliberations (Gillman *et al*, 1997: 190).

Why narrative research?

Stop and Think
The next question would seem to be why: why should therapists conduct narrative research? Give some thought now about why you as a therapist might conduct narrative research. Suggest a few possible benefits.

First, narratives are important in people's lives. Somers states:

> 'that stories guide action; that people construct identities (however multiple and changing) by locating themselves or being located within the repertoire of emplotted stories; that 'experience' is constituted through narratives; that people make sense of what has happened and is happening to them by attempting to assemble or in some way to integrate these happenings within one or more narratives; and that people are guided to act in certain ways and not others, on the basis of the projections, expectations, and memories derived from a multiple but ultimately limited repertoire of available social, public, and cultural narratives. (1994: 613–614)

Narrative approaches to understanding bring the researcher more closely into the investigative process than do quantitative and statistical methods. Through narrative, researchers come in contact with participants as people engaged in the process of interpreting themselves. Writing of her experiences using a life story approach in health care research, Smith states:

> Participants were seen to develop new insights into their personal experiences, family relationships, and social world understandings. They declared stronger feelings of self-value and personal rights; expressed increased confidence in the validity of their own perceptions; experienced greater integration of past events into their present sense of self; and presented an overall more centered, grounded, and self-cohering demeanor. (2000: 19)

Thompson, looking from the viewpoint of a historian, suggests that oral history sources in the history of health and welfare brings three special advantages (2000: 3–4). The first is that it contributes to a fuller and more comprehensive documenting of the lives of people of many kinds. Widdershoven and Smits emphasize the quality of the data provided by narratives:

> A narrative approach to ethical issues in health care focuses on the stories that participants tell about their experiences. These stories give us insight into motives, expectations, aims and convictions of the persons involved. A narrative can make us understand how people give meaning to a concrete situation and why they respond to it through a specific action. Narratives are not just descriptions of feelings and actions; they present these feelings and actions as part of a practice. (1996: 285–286)

In general terms the voices of less powerful groups within society are not present in historical writings. Hirsch writes:

> Since people with disabilities constitute one of the most powerless groups of individuals in any society, it is also not surprising that disability issues have not been broadly dealt with in historical writings ... the use of oral histories in disability studies could allow yet another group to find a voice, could lead to a new view of local and social history, and could help create a deeper understanding of cultural conditions which affect everyone. (1995: 1)

Likewise, in their review of different approaches to understanding and interpreting the history of learning difficulty, Walmsley and Atkinson argue that, 'those historians who have turned their attention to the subject have not recognized the political importance, or the value, of trying to access the perspectives of people with learning difficulties' (2000: 198). The same might be argued of the perspectives of practitioners in the history of the development of therapy.

The second advantage, as suggested by Thompson, is that it allows for the exploration of areas of life that written records scarcely touch. The third advantage is that oral sources can provide a basis for the re-examination of well-documented spheres through new perspectives.

Gillman (1999) says that narrative research aims to give voice to the silenced or subjugated stories of marginalized groups in society. Oral history has made its most striking contributions in Britain through community work, including the use of oral history in reminiscence therapy. There has been a strong and growing movement among social workers and health professionals working with older people for the use of memories of the past in group work. Stimulated by tape recordings, music, photographs and slides from the period of their childhood or youth – reminiscence therapy can restore an active interest in life to older people who have given up hope (Thompson, 2000). In general terms, oral history can be a significant resource for political groups and emergent social movements: in the women's movement; for trade unionists and working class communities; for immigrant and ethnic communities; and in gay and lesbian politics.

How is narrative research conducted?

> **Stop and Think**
> Narrative research is usually carried out through the medium of the interview. For this exercise, think of yourself as the research participant rather than the researcher. You are a participant in a research project to examine the 'career of therapy' from the viewpoint of the therapist. A narrative approach is being used in this research. What question might the researcher ask to elicit your story as a therapist?

Open-ended questions are used to generate extended accounts, for example 'tell me what happened when …', or 'were you ever in a situation like …?', or 'can you describe a time when you …?' These kinds of questions encourage the respondent to answer with a story. In addition, probe questions can be used to encourage the progression of the story, such as 'can you tell me more about that?' The interviewer needs to develop active listening skills, such as nodding, asking for clarification of a point, or summarizing to check his or her understanding of the story so far.

In their review of narrative approaches in therapy research, Larson and Fanchiang argue that these approaches 'provide the therapist with a view of the client's daily occupation routines, family member relationships, sociocultural influences, and the effects of these factors on the delivery of occupational therapy services ... The small narrative windows that occur daily in occupational therapy services can be important in situating a therapy episode into an ongoing life story' (1996: 249).

Bornat is clear about the effectiveness of interviews in data collection:

> To talk to people about working lives, domestic relationships, childhood, experiences of migration, racism, exclusions, free time and pleasures is to challenge historical and political orthodoxies. But it is also more than that, like other oral historians, I saw the interview as a source of data which was untarnished and more real than any other type of data that I had previously sought out. (1993: 85)

In her life history research with people with learning difficulties, Walmsley (1998) supported the interview process in a number of ways. She used 'life maps' and 'network diagrams'. A life map shows key points in an individual's life, and a network diagram depicts the people involved in a participant's social network. She also found that participants' photographs provided useful prompts.

It is essential that interviews are audio/video recorded and accurately transcribed so that the story can be depicted in a way that is faithful to the experience of the respondent. The issues of 'informed consent' and 'confidentiality' need to be carefully considered and discussed with the participant prior to the interview.

It is something of a convention for an oral history interview to progress chronologically through a person's life course, beginning with early childhood memories and then through the decades of life and the life events of, say, marriage, becoming a parent and so on. Bornat (1993), however, found that the memories of many of the old people she interviewed did not fall into such a neat chronological life course.

The relevance of narrative approaches for therapists

Using a life story approach in therapy research, Blanche emphasized the insights she gained to each client's background. She states: 'stereotyping persons and treating them as homogeneous ethnic or racial groups saves time but is not effective. Listening to a client's life story may give us information we need to place our services within the complexity of his or her life' (1996: 275).

Dominant ideas in professional practice, such as medical diagnosis and theories of rehabilitation, have the power to construe meaning and shape the attitudes and actions of therapists and their clients. Mattingly, discussing the clinical reasoning of occupational therapists suggests that '... general treatment goals derived from general knowledge of functional deficits and developmental possibilities were insufficient guides to practice' (1991: 1001). She asserts that therapists should understand the patient's experience of disability, injury and illness, and not just the technical details of impairment, in order to achieve therapeutic goals. In doing so, therapists can draw upon the listening and empathy skills they use in their clinical practice, and bridge the gap between research and practice.

There has also been a strong and growing interest among social workers and health professionals in reminiscence therapy, which involves working with groups of older people to stimulate memories of the past through the use of tape recordings, music and photographs of the period (Thompson, 2000). In addition, the compilation of life history books by collating information, photographs and documents from past homes, relatives and previous workers is also a well established therapeutic activity with groups such as children in foster care.

Narrative methods inform the domains of both therapy and research and embody practices which are familiar to therapists.

For example, Kohler Reissman suggests that researchers can bear witness to untellable stories:

> A primary way in which individuals make sense of their experience is by casting it in a narrative form. This is especially so of difficult life transitions and trauma. (1993: 4).

In a review of the therapy literature, Frank (1996) summarized the qualitative methods used by occupational therapists to accomplish the goals of clinical practice, as: making systematic observations; listening to patients' stories; validating interpretations they make about their patients' lives; and interacting and collaborating with patients to create new worlds, new meanings, and new life stories. She states: 'These methods all rely on a narrative approach – that is on telling a story' (1996: 251). Though there are few examples of narrative research in the physiotherapy literature, the issues that physiotherapists address in their work with clients can be similar. Illness, injury and impairment disrupt the life story that we envisage for ourselves, and most therapy clients have to come to terms with these altered meanings and their implications for identity.

Conclusion

The challenge is for therapists to play their part in the telling of stories. As Atkinson recognizes: 'Therapists are well placed, through their work and in their relationships with clients, to play an active part in the telling of stories. This starts with recognizing that everyone has a personal past, and acknowledging and respecting that past. It goes further: it means listening to the life story when it is told; helping where possible, with the telling and the researching of that story; and recording the present sensitively, so that today's stories are recorded for the future in ways that people themselves approve' (1999: 21).

We must, however, end with a note of caution. Narrative research is, of course, subject to the same ethical considerations as all other therapy research. Informed consent and confidentiality are essential. Though, as mentioned above, Smith (2000) came to very positive conclusions about life story research, she found it could be an emotionally fraught process. She states: 'Several women went through periods of emotional distress during the interviews, demonstrated by increased disorganization of their thoughts, unsteady voices, physical shaking and getting cold, increased nervous activity, becoming silent ...' (2000: 17). The researcher is responsible for anticipating back-up support for participants who become distressed during the research process. Narrative research should not be entered into under the illusion that it is an easy option. Stories are serious business.

Participatory approaches to research

with Maureen Gillman

What is a participatory approach?

This chapter addresses questions relating to power in research. Researchers and participants within research have increasingly raised issues of control: 'Who initiates? Who determines salient questions? Who determines what constitutes findings? Who determines how data will be collected? Who determines in what forms the findings will be made public, if at all? Who determines what representations will be made of participants in the research?' (Lincoln and Guba, 2000: 175). Research, it can be argued, is usually carried out by the powerful on the powerless and can be a source of maintaining or even exacerbating oppression (Oliver, 1992). People at the bottom of any hierarchy rarely have sufficient power to generate knowledge, indeed such power is usually held by those furthest from the situation. As Brechin states, 'Research tends to be owned and controlled by researchers, or by those who, in turn, own and control the researchers' (1993: 73).

Participatory methodologies have many historical roots. They tend to have arisen from qualitative research approaches which aim to reflect, explore and disseminate the views, concerns, feelings and experiences of research participants from their own perspectives. The realization of participatory research goes beyond this, however, to engage participants in the design, conduct and evaluation of research, with the construction of non-hierarchical research relations (Zarb, 1992). Participatory research, then, attempts to change the social relations of research processes. In feminist research (Olesen, 1998), research into ethnic concerns (Stanfield, 1998), in the field of social care (Kemshall and Littlechild, 2000) and disability issues (Zarb, 1992), some researchers have sought to engage in research which empowers rather than exploits people.

A crucial tenet of participatory research is that it is research *with* rather than on people (Reason, 1994) and research which puts 'the first last' (Chambers, 1997). The research process is viewed as a potential source of change and empowerment for the research participants as well as a process for influencing professional policy and practice by reflecting the views and opinions of service users. Reason and Heron (1986) believe that participatory research invites people to participate in the co-creation of knowledge about themselves. Using the term 'partnership research', Lloyd *et al* (1996) recognize similar principles: non-hierarchical research relationships in setting the research agenda, data analysis and dissemination.

Participatory research is an approach which has been evolving in recent years. There are a number of relevant approaches that claim to be essentially 'participatory', such as 'democratic research', 'participatory action research' and 'emancipatory action research'. Kemmis and McTaggart say of 'participatory action research' that it is a concept which is 'applied to a variety of research approaches employed in a diversity of fields and settings' (2000: 567). The general change in terminology from 'research subjects' to 'research participants' is indicative of the influence of participatory approaches. We would argue, with Cornwell and Jewkes, that 'the key difference between participatory and conventional methodologies lies in the location of power in the research process' (1995: 1667). At its most radical, participatory research aims to involve, at every stage of the research process (choice of topics, methods, evaluation and dissemination), those towards whom research is normally directed, people who Chambers (1997) describes as 'the last', for example rural village dwellers in developing countries, patients and disabled people.

When participatory research is seen as a shift in power in the process of research, it is possible to distinguish among different modes and degrees of participation:

- Consultative – People are asked for their opinions and consulted by researchers before interventions are made. Thus, for instance, an interview schedule is designed through consultation.
- Collaborative – Researchers and participants work together on projects designed, initiated and managed by researchers. Participants may act as participant observers.
- Collegiate – Researchers and participants work together as partners in the whole decision-making process of design, implementation and management (Cornwall and Jewkes, 1995).

Why use a participatory approach?

Stop and Think

Having begun by defining what is meant by 'participatory' approaches in research, the next obvious question is why? Think of a possible research project and suggest some reasons why you as a researcher might adopt a participatory approach.

de Koning and Martin offer two reasons why participatory approaches have grown in popularity. First, 'there is an increasing recognition of the gap between the concepts and models professionals use to understand and interpret reality and the concepts and perspectives of different groups in the community' (1996: 1). Second, 'many factors, cultural, historical, socio-economic and political, which are difficult to measure have a crucial influence on the outcomes of interventions and efforts to improve the health of people' (1996: 1). The following are some of the key features which are generally thought to characterize participatory research:

- It breaks down the mystique surrounding research.
- It ensures that the problems researched are perceived as problems by the community to which the research is directed.
- It helps to develop self-confidence, self-reliance and skills within people to whom the research is directed.
- It encourages democratic interaction and transfer of power to the research participants.

Participatory research, then, is essentially about establishing equality in research relationships, that is giving more say in research to people who are more usually subjected to research. In this way, too, issues of participation can be seen as closely related to ethical issues.

Knowledge is often put to use in ways which are not beneficial to the people to whom the research is directed. Research into the treatment of a particular disease, for example, may serve to maintain the status quo by failing to address the social, economic and political factors involved in its aetiology. At this point we shall refer to two examples of therapy research which not only attempted to move towards a participatory approach but also engaged in issues of shifting power. The first, from the field of physiotherapy, examined the views of users about the services they experienced as a result of stroke. Thomas and Parry, 1996 critically reflected on the shifting of power in favour of service users. They concluded that, 'incorporating collaborative partnerships into research designs can empower users by giving them the power and opportunity to influence generations of research-based knowledge that has impact on them' (1996: 12). They argue that there should be partnership at every stage with users having a role in designing research, validating findings, and identifying how to disseminate the research findings.

The second study, conducted by an occupational therapist, explored perceptions of quality of life among people with high spinal cord injuries. Hammell (2000) reflected on representation and accountability in her research. In relation to the former, she acknowledged that the choice of extracts from interviews used in subsequent reports was hers and reflected her priorities. Reviewing the literature addressing representation, she found 'far less attention has been paid to concerns of retaining the voices, perspectives and priorities of the participants in the phase of data analysis, writing up and subsequent publication' (2000: 66). Reflecting on accountability, she emphasized accountability to research participants. She proposed a number of questions researchers should ask themselves about their research, including:

- Who is likely to benefit from it?
- Who do we want to value our research?
- Does the research process reflect this?
- Will the research findings be published in formats accessible to those who are most likely to benefit from the information? (2000: 70)

Participatory approaches and emancipatory ideals

Perhaps the most controversial issue in the whole area of 'participatory approaches' is the notion that research can be emancipatory. Thompson summarizes 'emancipatory practice' as helping to set people free from:

- Discriminatory attitudes, values, actions and cultural assumptions.
- Structures of inequality and oppression, both within organizations and in the social order more broadly.
- The barriers of bad faith and alienation that stand in the way of empowerment and self-direction.
- Powerful ideological and other social forces that limit opportunities and maintain the status quo.
- Traditional practices which, although often based on good intentions, have the effect of maintaining inequalities and halting progress towards more appropriate forms of practice. (1998: 40–41).

Such ideals are most evident in notions of 'participatory action research', feminist approaches, and emancipatory research in disability studies. What place might they have in therapy research conducted by students and practitioners? We shall look first at the general stance and then take emancipatory research in disability studies as a particular example.

For Kemmis and McTaggart being emancipatory is a defining characteristic of participatory action research. It 'aims to help people recover, and release themselves, from the constraints of irrational, unproductive, unjust, and unsatisfying social structures that limit their self-development and self-determination' (2000: 597). Research which espouses emancipatory ideals is decidedly and overtly political. Participatory action research goes beyond participation in research processes to engage in the transformation of reality and to overcome 'irrationality, injustice, alienation and suffering' (2000: 592).

In the area of disability, it can be argued that emancipatory research, unlike participatory research, is not a research methodology as such, but rather part of the struggle of disabled people to control the decision-making processes that shape their lives and to achieve full citizenship. As Barton states: 'The task of changing the social relations and conditions of research production is to be viewed as part of the wider struggle to remove all forms of oppression and discrimination in the pursuit of an inclusive society' (1998:38).

Emancipatory research goes further than participatory research by aiming to change the social relations of research production, with disabled people taking complete control of the research process. In emancipatory research the social relations of research production are conceived as part of the processes of changing society to ensure the full participation of disabled people. Barnes explains:

> Emancipatory research is about the systematic demystification of the structures and processes which create disability and the establishment of a workable 'dialogue' between the research community and disabled people in order to facilitate the latter's empowerment. To do this researchers must learn how to put their knowledge and skills at the disposal of disabled people. (1992: 122)

It can be argued that participatory and emancipatory approaches focus on different processes of social change. Engagement in participatory research is, ostensibly, a process of empowerment whereby individuals are enabled to take control over their own lives (including participation in research). Emancipatory research is directed towards liberation from institutional discrimination by the elimination of structural, environmental and attitudinal barriers that marginalize disabled people and prevent them from leading full and active lives (Swain *et al*, 1998). In emancipatory research, the production of research is part of the liberation of disabled people, that is part of the process of changing society to ensure full participative citizenship. This is research conceived as political action in which the processes and products are the tools of disabled people in the achievement of their liberation. Emancipatory research is not necessarily qualitative. For instance, emancipatory research into the housing stock and, in particular, accessibility of housing for disabled people is likely to take the form of a quantitative survey to produce statistics to influence housing policies. Zarb sums up the fundamental difference between participatory and emancipatory research as follows:

> Participatory research which involves disabled people in a meaningful way is perhaps a prerequisite to emancipatory research in the sense that researchers can learn from disabled people and vice versa, and that it paves the way for researchers to make themselves 'available' to disabled people – but it is no more than that. Simply increasing participation and involvement will never by itself constitute emancipatory research unless and until it is disabled people themselves who are controlling the research and deciding who should be involved and how. (1992: 128)

Participatory and emancipatory are, therefore, two distinct, though by no means incompatible, research paradigms. As Stalker (1998) suggests, there are shared 'beliefs' within the two paradigms, but we believe that the differences also need to be recognized. In particular, beginner researchers can engage in participatory approaches and to do so, in our experience, can enhance even the most small-scale projects. A project in which clients are interviewed, for instance, is more likely to address the clients' agendas and concerns if a participatory approach is used in designing the interview schedule. Claims that research is emancipatory are, however, problematic for even the most experienced of researchers, though emancipatory ideals can offer a basis for researchers to reflect on who benefits from their research. In terms of emancipatory intentions, a key question is: does the research support research participants in their struggle against oppression and the removal of barriers to equal opportunities and a full participatory democracy for all?

Strategies for participatory approaches

> **Stop and Think**
> Having considered what participatory approaches are and why they might be adopted in research, the next question is how. Take some time now to consider strategies for achieving a more participatory approach in practice. To do this you might select a project you know or are planning and make a list of all you or the researcher might do to involve research participants as co-researchers.

Any research method can be used, but the emphasis is on those which are eclectic, inventive and flexible, giving room for new ideas to emerge and allowing for changes of plan and direction as the research proceeds. Methods are adapted to suit the particular situation and the people involved, rather than squeezing ideas into a fixed method. With traditional research, complex issues are sometimes simplified or avoided because the methods are too rigid to accommodate them. With the participatory approach, as Cornwall and Jewkes state, 'research activities are expanded to encompass performance, art and story-telling, as well as conventional methods such as focus group discussions' (1995: 1671).

You might have mentioned the involvement of research participants in every aspect and at every stage within a research project. We have been involved in research projects which have adopted the following strategies.

- Research participants, or representatives, can be involved in the steering groups which oversee the planning and development of the whole project.
- Open-ended interviews seem to give participants more power in determining what is talked about and what is not. Where more structured methods are used, participants can be involved in deciding on the questions to be asked.
- In some projects it can be possible to involve participants in data collection, e.g. in recording their observations or interviewing other participants.
- Researchers can go back to participants with tentative findings, and refine them in the light of participants' reactions. This is a way of involving participants in the analysis of findings, sometimes called respondent-validation.

One aim of participatory research is to provide educational opportunities to those who are so often at the receiving end of research directed by 'experts'. This, it is hoped, will have the effect of increasing their skills, self-reliance and self-confidence, leading to social action which they perceive to be relevant. People are generally more committed if they take part in activities rather than being passive recipients; the researchers will also have much to learn from this approach.

Reflective practice and participatory practitioner research

As Shaw (2000) suggests, notions of participation can be found in different forms of inquiry including, as we shall discuss here, participatory reflective inquiry and practice. The traditional model of professional development has separated theory from practice and perpetuates their separation. In more recent years, however, this has been broken down through the notion of 'reflective inquiry and practice' which has been encompassed within and propagated through widespread developments in professional training.

Therapists can connect with the participatory paradigm through the notions of reflective practice and practitioner research. Reflective practice is the capacity of a therapist to think, talk or write about a piece of practice with the intention to review new meanings or perspectives on the situation. At a personal level it can help therapists to examine the beliefs and values they bring to their practice for signs of stereotypical thinking or prejudice. At a professional level it can provide a framework for evaluating theories and models of practice in terms of their potential to oppress or marginalize people. Such reflection can help therapists to construct models of practice informed by notions of social justice and based on collaboration and partnership with clients. It also provides an opportunity to prioritize the issues and concerns of patients as topics for research. Practitioner research should be 'designed so as to give a say to all participants' and 'involves trying to see things from the perspective of the patients or clients' (Reed and Biott, 1995: 195).

Practitioner research is concerned with issues and problems that arise in practice and it aims to bring about change, or influence policy in the practice arena. Some common concerns investigated by researcher/practitioners include: deficiencies in services or resources, conflict between professional values and agency requirements, and the improvement of practice. Practitioner research provides a framework for formulating practice knowledge and allows such knowledge to be disseminated to other professionals. Many of the skills and competencies associated with practice are transferable to the conduct of participatory research. Therapists are educated to engage with clients in a respectful and meaningful way, and to encourage patients to express themselves.

Practitioner reflexivity is just as central to the conduct of research as it is to practice. Indeed, Schon suggests that practice and research are inextricably linked through the process of reflection. 'When someone reflects-in-action he (sic) becomes a researcher in the practice context' (1993: 20). Adopting a reflective approach to research allows the therapist to question the power relations of research and influences the process at each stage. Fook argues that:

A reflective approach affirms the importance of experiential and interconnected ways of knowing the world and favours more emancipatory and participatory research practices. (1996: 5)

Practitioner research is grounded in the everyday world of practice and can reflect the voices of stakeholders in that context. To be of value, research does not have to be large scale or 'scientific' in the positivist tradition. Methods such as 'case study' and 'life history' are familiar territory for therapists and have the potential to be more participatory than those methods which do not give patients or clients a voice. All research has the potential to exploit and oppress participants if attention is not paid to the power imbalances between researchers and research participants. The participatory paradigm represents an overarching framework for informing the conduct and evaluating the products of practitioner research.

Though reflective inquiry and practice can incorporate participatory principles, it is important to recognize that, as we have emphasized in this chapter, research differs in terms of the form and degree of participation. Indeed, as Shaw recognizes, 'Schon does not seem to envisage any directly participative dimension. His examples focus extensively on the practitioner in discussion with colleagues and supervisors, rather than involving students, children or other service users' (2000: 30–31). Participation, like emancipation, can be seen as an ideal for evaluating and reflecting on the process of research. The following two projects are examples of practitioner research which prioritize the voices of clients, though the control of the research process remains essentially with the practitioners.

Martlew (1996), a physiotherapist, evaluated on-site physiotherapy in a day hospice providing care for patients with terminal illness, using 'client-centred action research'. She concluded that the learning experience was 'greater because this study was conducted by a practitioner-researcher doing her own action research' and that 'this study has confirmed the benefit of taking time to listen sensitively – both for the professionals, to gain greater insight into patient problems, hopefully leading to more appropriate and therefore effective intervention; and for patients who feel supported and understood' (1996: 564).

Blanche (1996), an occupational therapist, explored the effect of cultural differences on the delivery of health care services through a life story approach with the mother of a disabled child. She used a 'co-operative story making' approach which rejects the ideology of 'observed versus observer' and sees both the interviewer and the informer as building the story together. She concludes that: 'clinicians need to acknowledge the client's and their own culture as well as the perceptions, expectations, values, and beliefs that are inherent in each ... Stereotyping persons and treating them as homogeneous ethnic or racial groups saves time but is not effective. Listening to a client's life story may give us the information we need to place our services within the complexity of his or her life' (1996: 174–275).

Client-centred practice may provide a foundation for participatory practitioner research. However, 'professional status is derived from a number of sources of power which fundamentally remain unchallenged by professionally led initiatives to increase service-user participation' (Braye, 2000: 17).

Conclusion

Participatory research may seem somewhat removed from the everyday world of the practising therapist, but this need not be so. A central theme of this approach is that practically everyone is capable of contributing to the research effort. Therapists, therapy assistants and clients may be reluctant to become involved in research, believing that enormous expertise is required and that it is best left in the capable hands of the 'experts'. Although it is true that some knowledge of research methodology is helpful, therapists and their clients are at the sharp end of clinical practice and the knowledge they have gained through years of experience should never be underestimated or thought to be inferior to that of experienced researchers. Therapists are also in a position to involve people who are often researched but who are rarely consulted. Participatory research is a democratic means of accelerating social change and reducing exploitation through the empowerment of research participants. In developing processes of critical reflection, however, questions need to be raised about the mechanisms and processes required to facilitate and sustain participation (Kemshall and Littlechild, 2000b: 239–240).

- What type of participation is being sought and why; who is to participate, how and why?
- How can participation by hidden and marginalized groups be actively sought and maintained?
- How can the differing interests and expectations of those involved (researchers, participants, funders) be balanced and negotiated?
- What are the mechanisms to facilitate 'activeness' and the likelihood of participants' control over implementation?
- Who has ownership, use and publication of research material?

Any therapist engaged in participatory research will need to reflect on these issues.

Action research and clinical audit

There are increasing pressures within the NHS for practice to be grounded in evidence and to be demonstrably effective. For therapists who are interested in carrying out local projects with the aim of directly benefiting patients and users of services, action research may offer a meaningful strategy (Denscombe, 1998). Clinical audit shares many characteristics with action research (Birkett, 1995) and provides therapists with evidence about the quality and effectiveness of practice. The research understanding and skills acquired through studying this and other books will help therapists to gather reliable and valid audit data, as well as to participate in more formal research enquiries.

Action research

Action research describes a broad strategy of research and does not entail particular research designs or methods. Case studies, interviews, questionnaires, observation and experiment may all provide relevant data for an action research project. It is a strategy that can be applied to a range of health, education, and community development issues. So what characterizes this approach to research?

- Action research is directed at implementing a change in *one's own* practice and self-critically evaluating its effects.
- It deals with a local, practical issue affecting either a small group, larger organization or community.
- It seeks to develop a deep understanding of how the process of change affects all participants, and so aims to develop a theoretical perspective.
- Although context-specific, some generalization may be possible because a detailed understanding of the change process and the effects of intervention are developed throughout the project.

An example of action research will clarify these points. Hart & Bond (1995) described how changes to medication routines were implemented in a residential home for elderly people. Initial observations by the new manager had revealed many examples of poor practice. The process of dispensing medication was not rigorous, there was conflicting information about prescribed dosage in some patients' notes and some GPs were offering many repeat prescriptions without monitoring residents' health. A wide-ranging programme of staff development was introduced, which included the care workers' own ideas for improved practice. Information was also gathered from consultations with GPs and local pharmacists. The effects, in terms of changes in dispensing practice, and staff attitudes to standards of care, were assessed in many different ways over many months. The reflective awareness stimulated by this programme led to care staff instigating 'spin-off' projects, for example, to reduce laxative use through improving the residents' nutrition, and to develop improved care of residents with visual impairments. The effects of these changes on residents' health was not documented but clearly could have been assessed in a longer project.

Several features of action research emerge from this example. Firstly, action research traditionally follows a cycle (or spiral) of phases (Hart & Bond, 1995). See Figure 18.1.

This sequence mirrors the clinical process of assessing clients' needs, formulating a suitable response or intervention, and reviewing progress. Each phase may be lengthy. Secondly, action research projects are commonly multi-layered, both in the inter-

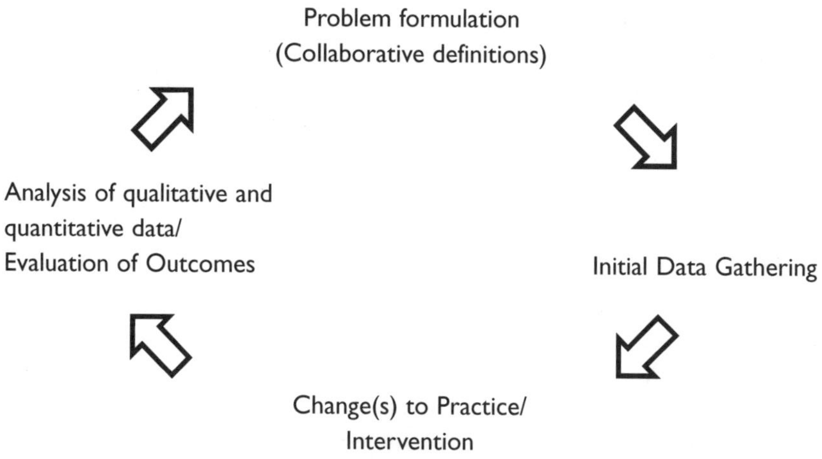

Problem formulation
(Collaborative definitions)

Analysis of qualitative and
quantitative data/
Evaluation of Outcomes

Initial Data Gathering

Change(s) to Practice/
Intervention

Figure 18.1 The cycle of action research

vention itself and in the data collected. Because a change to practice is introduced, the design commonly has quasi-experimental
features (see Chapter 11). The evaluation often draws upon
both objective data (such as doses of medication or number of
GP consultations) and more qualitative data (such as agendas
from staff meetings, and field notes of observed staff interac-
tions). It is nevertheless possible to carry out a smaller action
research project investigating the outcomes of a change in
therapy or care practice with a more limited set of data. Thirdly,
action research projects often continue for many months as the
various stages of initial data-gathering, change and evaluation take
time to complete. Fourthly, implemented changes can have negative as well as positive effects. The project described above is
not unusual in encountering some initial staff resentment about
the changes to care practices. It is useful for action researchers
to have some knowledge of social/organizational theory in order
to monitor and understand these aspects of the change process.

Action research usually also aspires to being non-hierarchical
and non-exploitative. Instead of having a marked division
between researchers and participants, all may be regarded as
co-researchers with different forms of expertise that will
enhance the project. As far as possible, each participant in the
change process (whether staff or client) is encouraged to

contribute to every phase of the research project, including putting forward ideas for needed changes to practice, and identifying appropriate measures for evaluating the outcomes. However, some authors (such as Hart & Bond, 1995) note that this ideal may not be attained in all action research, and needs to be the subject of critical reflection. For example, if the research is carried out in a setting that suffers from high staff turnover and discontent, participants may drop out or even sabotage the implementation of change. Also change itself risks alienating some staff. A project that seeks to empower clients may in turn be experienced by staff as disempowering. Action researchers need to have an even higher level of sensitivity to interpersonal issues than is usually required in more conventional research.

Various types of action research have been suggested, each with rather distinctive values and objectives (Hart & Bond, 1995). Of particular relevance to occupational therapists and physiotherapists are the 'professionalizing' and 'empowering' forms of project. Professionalizing action research has the principal aim of enhancing reflective practice and professional control over work. The approach is particularly well suited to exploring therapists' clinical reasoning processes in a way that combines research with staff development (e.g. Mattingly & Gillette, 1991). Empowering action research tends to be community-based, involving service users or vulnerable groups, and seeks to promote 'voice'. Whilst paid staff may initially provide accommodation and perhaps the impetus for meetings, they will then work to hand over influence and control to the users themselves. The users are likely to evaluate the effects of the change process directly and identify further strategies for meeting their own needs. Further information on emancipatory and participatory research is found in Chapter 17.

It is possible for an action research phase to follow on from a more traditional research study. To illustrate, let us assume that a conventionally scientific randomized controlled trial demonstrates the benefits of an exercise intervention for reducing falls among elderly people. A professionalizing phase of action research could then follow. Therapists might participate in the following:

- Discuss the implications of the findings for professional practice.
- Critically evaluate existing health promotion advice to clients.
- Devise a new health promotion intervention that aims to increase exercise among elderly clients.
- Meet regularly to share good practice.
- Determine what data should be collected to evaluate the outcomes.
- Evaluate the outcomes in consultation with clients (and the outcomes for therapists also).
- Instigate further changes in practice if necessary.

An 'empowering' phase may also be appropriate. This could for example involve elderly residents in sheltered accommodation in discussing the evidence about falls, consulting with them to determine their interests in physical activity and to explore their preferred ways of increasing activity (change stage). If an empowering approach is taken, the residents may themselves arrange further meetings to monitor the benefits and difficulties that they encounter in building more physical activity into their lives (evaluation stage).

Action research presents a number of challenges. Complex sets of quantitative and qualitative data can be difficult to analyse and synthesize. Mattingly & Gillette (1991) describe the challenge of analysing over 2000 pages of field notes and transcripts, as well as 30 videotapes of clinical sessions. Whilst 'insider' researchers are usually more sensitive to the dynamics of an organization, they also risk bias and a lack of objectivity. Participant observation (e.g. of team meetings) raises ethical difficulties, and power differentials may continue to exert unhealthy influence within the research 'team' (Uzzell, 1995). Action research tends to provide a complex local case study the findings of which may, therefore, be difficult to generalize. Nevertheless, when well managed, it can stimulate empowerment among both service providers and users, ownership of change and a self-critical, reflective approach to practice.

Stop and Think

A team of therapists wishes to incorporate more health promotion into their interventions with patients experiencing back pain, and evaluate the effectiveness of this intervention. One therapist suggests carrying out a randomized controlled trial with two groups: one randomly selected group of patients receiving a 10 minute 'healthy lifestyle' consultation with a supporting leaflet, in addition to the 'usual' intervention, and the control group receiving only the usual intervention. The therapist suggests measuring patients' knowledge about recommended health behaviours as the dependent variable.

Another therapist suggests setting up an *action research* project in this field.

1. Outline in basic terms how you might achieve and evaluate a health promotion intervention through an action research strategy.
2. Determine two or three differences between your action research plan and the conventional research outlined above.
3. Find one advantage and one disadvantage in your action research approach compared with the traditional research outlined above.

In the above exercise, it is likely that you will have suggested an extensive *consultation process* with clients to determine their perceived needs – for information, exercise facilities, family support and so on. The intervention *may* then be tailored to meet individual needs (e.g. the health promotion needs of a young father may be very different from that of an isolated elderly woman, so a single leaflet for all may not be appropriate). You might have considered adopting an *empowering* strategy, for example encouraging clients to advocate for local environmental change to improve health (e.g. tackle congested roads filled with traffic fumes; campaign for a direct bus route to the local park). The intervention will almost certainly include *reflective self-appraisal* by staff – what are their barriers to incorporating health promotion interventions, or adopting healthier personal lifestyles? Do they see themselves as role models for patients? In evaluating the change in practice, the effects of increasing health awareness could be monitored not only with clients but within the team – since the start of the project, are staff more aware of their own diet, exercise and stress management strategies? Organizational practices which jeopardize therapists' health (such as expectations that staff will work across lunch-breaks) may also be tackled. Evaluation of outcomes may lead to additional changes to practice. For example, if evaluation shows that clients have quite good knowledge of healthy behaviour but limited awareness of local facilities such as parks and swimming pools, then this additional information may be made available.

The main advantage of the action research strategy is in the depth of information collected, which provides for more sensitive intervention and evaluation opportunities. At its best, its non-hierarchical ethos can capture the commitment of everyone involved. It can mobilize the whole team to think deeply about health issues and reflect on practice. A key disadvantage is the size of the project and its rather open-ended nature. The outcomes are more difficult to quantify and will take longer to assess. Another disadvantage is that despite the richness of the information collected, the action research strategy does not fit comfortably within the dominant research culture of the NHS which accepts the randomized controlled trial as the 'gold standard'. Nevertheless, the NHS places great emphasis on quality assurance, and requires, through audit, evidence that services are effective and efficient. Action research is based on client-centred values and has much in common with high quality clinical audit. These features may lead action research to become more prominent in the future.

Clinical audit

Audit was introduced with other reforms of the NHS in 1989, in order to provide evidence of the effectiveness of professional interventions, and to improve the quality of services within resource constraints. 'Audit is a cyclical activity involving system-atic review of practice, identification of problems, development of possible solutions, implementation of changes and further review' (Green 1997: 384).

Although some authors (such as Barnard & Hartigan, 1998; the College of Occupational Therapists, 1998; and Sealey, 1999) make a distinction between 'clinical audit' and 'research', a defini-tion such as this shows clinical audit to have many features in common with action research (Birkett, 1995). Both types of study are:

- Concerned with evaluating practice and improving the effec-tiveness of services.
- Context-specific and shaped by professional and/or 'insider' concerns.
- Determined by a perceived local problem in the service or a recently implemented change to the service.
- Progressed through a cycle or spiral of tasks.

Nevertheless, clinical audit is usually a more circumscribed process, aims to gather a narrower set of data and makes much less claim to being participatory (although staff and user involve-ment is recommended, for example, by COT, 1998). Audit data can also provide evidence within a larger, more conventional research project. It may or may not contribute to theory devel-opment, depending upon the complexity of the problem being investigated. The same holds for action research. Some action research clearly develops theoretical understanding (e.g. Mattingly & Gillette, 1991) whereas other projects focus more on solving a complex problem (e.g. the example given by Hart & Bond, 1995).

The key feature of clinical audit, that distinguishes the endeav-our from other forms of enquiry, is that current practice is com-pared with recommended standards. Standards may be formulated by international bodies (such as the World Health Organization), national frameworks (such as the Patients' Charter), professional bodies (such as COT, CSP) or by clinicians at local Trust or Unit level (Barnard & Hartigan, 1998). Where possible, they are based on published evidence about effective practice that has been accumulated from research studies, but all

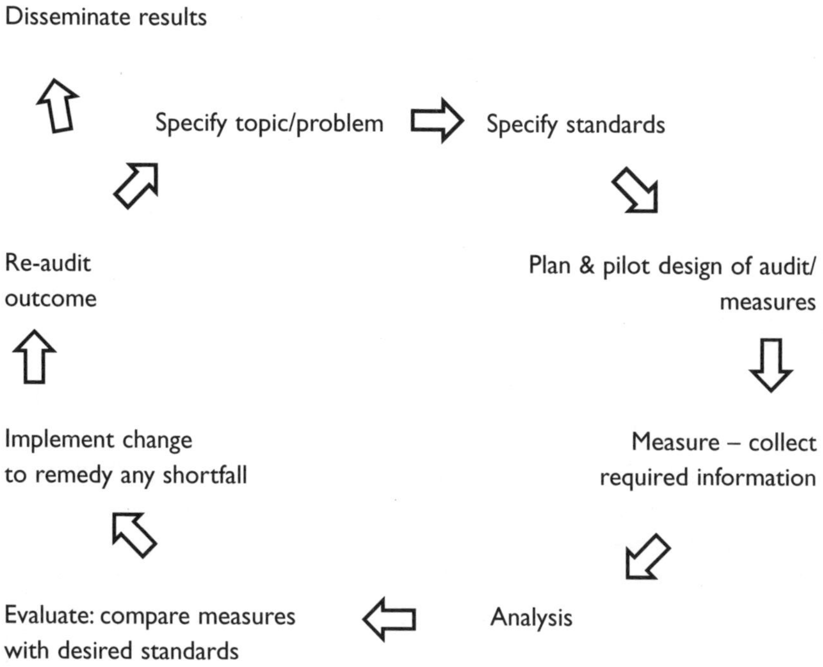

Disseminate results

      Specify topic/problem   ⇨ Specify standards

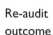   ⬂

Re-audit   Plan & pilot design of audit/
outcome   measures

⇧   ⬇

Implement change   Measure – collect
to remedy any shortfall   required information

⬃   ⬀

Evaluate: compare measures   ⇦   Analysis
with desired standards

Figure 18.2 The audit cycle (or spiral)
(Adapted from COT, 1998; Maggs, 1995; Sealey, 1999)

too often the evidence is lacking. Standards may relate to different areas of health care, broadly distinguished as structure/organization, process and outcome (Donabedian, 1992). Organizational (or structural) standards may refer, for example, to safe staffing levels, cleanliness of the environment or waiting list length. Process standards set out expectations for assessment, treatment and evaluation. For example, a particular intervention may be recommended for patients with a certain condition, or a specified number of treatment sessions may be set as standard. Outcome standards set out expectations concerning patients' responses to treatment. Different standards may be formulated for different groups of patients (Barnard, 1995). For some conditions, such as hip replacement, most patients will be expected to make a good recovery. With other conditions, such as multiple sclerosis, a successful outcome cannot be judged in terms of recovery. Maintained function or in-dependence in specified tasks may be set as outcome standards.

Once the standard(s) to which the service aspires have been set, auditors then need to determine the criteria by which per-formance will be judged. Measurable indicators of service quality must be identified. Degree of functional recovery and patient sat-isfaction provide examples of outcome indicators. As in any research study, the selected measures must have demonstrable validity and reliability, whether objective or subjective data are sought.

Stop and Think

Dobson (1995) reported an audit of the quality and effec-tiveness of physiotherapy for knee conditions. The time between patients' referral to the physiotherapy unit and their first consultation with the physiotherapist was taken as the measure of service quality. Find one advantage and one disadvantage of this measure.

Advantages of the measure include its reliability, and its availabil-ity within existing documentation. However, as a measure of service quality, 'waiting time' has disadvantages. 'Quality' includes more than delay to first appointment, so the measure has uncer-tain validity, and may lack sensitivity. A speedy appointment system does not guarantee skilful assessment and treatment. Also, patients' views were not considered. For example, it remains unknown whether patients prefer to wait a little longer for treatment in order to receive a more informative consulta-tion. Outcomes may be audited through measures designed specifically for the project or through use of standardized scales. Assessment methods include:

● Standardized scales: many reliable, validated scales are avail-able in published research/audit literature. For example, out-comes of interventions for patients with rheumatoid arthritis may be assessed through the AIMS (Arthritis Impact Measurement Scale). The COT (1998) resource pack lists many such standardized scales. If used prior to treatment to obtain baseline measures and again afterwards, changes in scores can contribute evidence about treatment effectiveness.

- Achievement of individualized treatment goals (e.g. Eames, Ward & Siddons, 1999).
- Review of information in case notes or treatment records (e.g. Dobson, 1995).
- Review of existing documentation (e.g. home visit assessment reports).
- Specifically designed questionnaires (e.g. patient satisfaction scales).

If designing a questionnaire specifically for the audit, its construction needs to pass through all the checks that have been recommended in Chapter 8 as vital for achieving a reliable, valid research questionnaire. For example, ambiguous or leading questions must be avoided and response instructions need to be clear. All audit measures need to be piloted to ensure clarity and acceptability to respondents (Barnard & Hartigan, 1998; Sealey, 1999). If the audit tools are not valid, apparently poor outcomes may reflect measurement error rather than service inadequacies. Advice about audit measures and analysis can usually be obtained from specialized audit departments within NHS Trusts, and also from the NCCA (National Centre for Clinical Audit, 1997).

Audit data may be collected retrospectively (from existing, previously collected material such as case-notes). However, where the data were not originally collected for audit purposes, they are likely to be incomplete. Alternatively, the audit may adopt a prospective design, using agreed measures, which are more likely to be relevant and useable.

As audit attempts to document the 'usual service' to patients, and is carried out by the professionals involved in the service, scrutiny by an ethics committee is not usually required. However, questionnaires, or other measures, that are introduced specifically for audit purposes may require ethics clearance, especially if vulnerable groups are involved (such as terminally ill patients or people with learning disabilities).

As explored earlier in the book (Chapter 4), good research generally depends upon a carefully thought out project proposal. Equally, with clinical audit, very detailed planning is required to determine appropriate standards, measurable criteria, dissemination strategies and possible future action on the basis of the findings. As in the action research examples described earlier, audit can be thwarted by professional resistance to implied criticism and an associated reluctance to implement the necessary changes (Redfern & Norman, 1996). The full audit cycle needs to be completed. This includes making changes in the service to rectify any shortfall between measured outcomes and standards and a re-audit to check that these changes have been successful (Sealey, 1999). A thorough clinical audit generally requires commitment by staff to evaluating their own practice. As with action research projects, willing and interested participation in audit can provide not only quality assurance to patients but a valuable means of critical self-appraisal, and continuing professional development for therapists. It also relies on, and develops, sound research skills.

Clinical audit as research

Some authors argue that clinical audit is not a form of research (Barnard & Hartigan, 1998; COT, 1998; Sealey, 1999). However, the authors appear to equate 'research' too narrowly with the experimental method. As this book illustrates, there is a wide variety of research methods and philosophies other than the randomized controlled treatment trial. 'Research tests new knowledge and methods of treatment, accounting for all possible variables, while clinical audit looks at what actually happens in a specific setting ...' (Barnard & Hartigan, 1998: 29). Leaving aside the issue of whether even experimental research can ever account for 'all' possible variables, this argument appears to discount qualitative explorations of patients' illness experiences, surveys of attitudes, and case studies as legitimate forms of research. Not all research examines cause and effect in the positivistic tradition. Qualitative researchers generally accept that people respond to their interpretations of events rather than to the objective nature of the event. Audit which gathers information about patients' satisfaction or unmet needs has much in common with other forms of survey research. Barnard & Hartigan (1998) also argue that 'research' focuses on knowledge whereas 'audit' focuses on the patients' experiences. This again seems to set up an artificial contrast, and ignores the many small-scale research studies which have a patient-centred (or person-centred) focus, such as studies of people adapting to long-term illness or impairment (e.g. Seymour, 1998).

Whilst some audits focus on very local, atheoretical issues (such as whether all patients receive appointments within a specified time) there are many examples of clinical audits which contribute to wider research in a field. For example, McIntyre (1999) showed how audit findings can both confirm existing research evidence and suggest the need for further, perhaps larger-scale psychosocial research. She described an audit of medical and occupational therapy case notes which revealed that falls were a common factor in the first admission of elderly people to a day hospital. Many psychosocial problems were discovered to follow on from a fall experience. There was a common loss of confidence and mobility following a fall, with 13% becoming housebound, and 59% becoming more dependent on family, friends and services. The results of the audit confirmed previous research into falling and suggested the need for interventions which reduce anxiety, build confidence and minimize dependence.

Research studies in health care settings often make use of audit findings as one strand of the data collected. For example, Tyson & Turner reported on the Southampton Stroke Audit. 'Uniquely, the audit not only examined the details of patient management and any inadequacies in the care, but also established the factors preventing optimum management' (1999: 227). This description shows that the enquiry was not only concerned to document any shortfall in services but also to establish possible reasons (or causal factors). This study clearly straddles audit and research, in supplementing the audit of professional notes with a patient satisfaction questionnaire, and a staff opinion survey to explore how staff accounted for service shortfalls. Staff expressed concern that the medical emphasis on rapid discharge hindered their attempts to help patients return to their former roles and valued occupations. The comprehensive results carry implications for service improvement elsewhere and suggest further research enquiry into the limiting effects of a biomedical perspective on rehabilitation processes.

Conclusion

Action research and clinical audit represent broad strategies of enquiry rather than specific methods. They share a focus on practical problem-solving, and evaluating the effects of changes in practice. Action research is usually set up as a highly collaborative enquiry, and therapists are also less likely to regard the audit process as onerous and time-consuming if they experience 'ownership' of the project. Commitment to changes recommended on the basis of action research or audit is enhanced when all professionals have been involved from the planning stage onwards. Both forms of enquiry can encourage critical reflection on practice and enhance professional development, as well as promoting more effective treatment and a more responsive service.

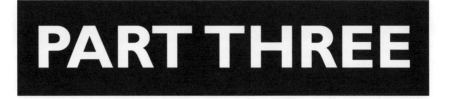

PART THREE

REPORTING AND DISSEMINATING RESEARCH FINDINGS

The writing process

The writing up of research can take a number of forms basically distinguished by the purpose of the report and the intended audience. There are three main categories of research report, though they are not necessarily separate:

1. Research reports written for examination or assessment purposes
The audience here of course is the marker or examiner, and the purpose for the student is the successful completion of the course requirements. This often takes the form of a research thesis.

2. Research reports written for feedback purposes
The audience here is those directly involved in the research, this can include research participants, institutions where the research took place, the steering committee, ethics committee and any organizations financing the research. This can include interim and final reports.

3. Research reports written to disseminate findings to a wider audience
This can include therapists, policy makers, other professionals and service providers, and mainly takes the form of publications in professional and academic journals.

In this chapter we shall look at the general principles of writing up research, particularly as they apply to a dissertation or thesis. In the next chapter we focus specifically on dissemination.

> **Stop and Think**
> Write down five images or ideas that you associate with the words 'writing up'.
> Write down three feelings that are triggered by the words 'writing up'.

We have found that, for some students, writing up is the most daunting part of the whole research process. Some students can avoid starting writing up and for some writing can feel like an exposure of themselves – their thinking and understanding made public. Alasuutari provides a good starting point for thinking about writing up:

> Writing is first and foremost analysing, revising and polishing the text. The idea that one produces ready-made text right away is just about as senseless as the cyclist who has never had to restore his or her balance. (1995: 178)

Though everyone has an individual way of working, it is our experience that writing up should not be thought of as the last stage of the research process. It is best conceived as a continuous process which builds throughout rather than being left until the end. This will allow you to make the best use of your supervisor, to engage with ideas and develop your thinking through writing: which is why the title of this chapter is *The Writing Process*.

The following guidelines adapted from Bell (1999) may provide a good starting point for working out your writing plan.

Acquire a good knowledge of word-processing
The computer, and in particular, word processing has changed the whole business of writing up, or at least the technical side of writing. The process of writing and redrafting has been transformed by the capacity to 'cut and paste' on the screen, saving earlier drafts. Furthermore the presentation of your writing up is important whatever the purposes of the report. The presentation of graphs, tables and other figures has been simplified by word-processing, though basic principles still apply. For instance,

the presentation of results should be succinct and clear, and graphics should only be used when necessary and should be presented as simply as possible (for example three-dimensional diagrams are rarely necessary). Most programmes have a spell-check, a grammar-check, a thesaurus; can format text such as by bullet points and numbered lists; insert tables; and even create contents pages. With compatibility between programmes, developments in technology have also facilitated co-authoring. For instance, drafts can be sent to a co-author or supervisor by e-mail. Speedy turn round can keep all the participants engaged in the process and encourage the flow of ideas.

Set deadlines/a timetable for writing up
This may well be required of you as part of a research proposal and deadlines can be set in discussion with your supervisor, whilst recognizing that some flexibility will be required.

Write regularly
As supervisors and students ourselves, we have found that supervision which is effective from both sides centres on work produced by the student. Furthermore, regular engagement in the writing process helps to keep the issues in mind, stimulates thinking and revision of key arguments.

Write up sections as you progress through your investigation
Some sections will be ready for at least a first draft of writing up before others. Many students we have worked with have begun the process of writing up with the methodology chapter, as much of their initial thinking and planning contributes to this chapter. Others start with the literature review and progress through the chapters in order.

Publicize your plans
As Bell (1999) suggests, telling friends and family about your writing routine can help in maintaining time periods for you to devote to writing. With many therapists, we have found, however, that it is pressures from work that can prevent the meeting of writing up deadlines. These are more difficult to counter and will depend on your circumstances. If your NHS Trust or manager

can see clinical value in getting the project written up and dis-seminated, possibly some time may be granted to you for the task.

Some processes and principles

The process of writing covers a number of activities including: finding ideas or planning; gathering information; synthesizing ideas; finding a structure; writing early drafts; reading text; nego-tiating feedback; writing later drafts; and editing. As French and Sim state:

> Writing takes time and patience, perseverance and mental stamina. It does not, however, require extraordinary talent, cre-ativity or expertise and is something every therapist can do. (1993: 22)

Bannister *et al* (1994: 162) emphasize that writing is a process of communication: 'Always keep in mind that the main point of a write-up ... is to communicate clearly your findings to others, to share your understandings of your results, to tell others what has possibly been learnt from your particular piece of research.' They suggest that you should aim for 'replicability', that is pre-senting sufficient information for the reader to be able to repeat your study if they so wish. Similarly in presenting interpretations of your findings you should attempt to present sufficient infor-mation for readers to see the basis of your reasoning and, ideally, to be able to come to their own alternative interpretations.

The use of English and writing style are also important and can be crucial in terms of the marks students receive for their work. Some common errors can detract the reader, such as problems with singular and plural words, for example 'data were collected' rather than 'data was collected'. Mistakes are also commonly made with pronouns, for instance 'the participant was asked for their opinion' should read either 'the participant was asked for his or her opinion' or 'the participants were asked for their opin-ions'. Burnard, also, lists some principles for writing a literature review that are generally applicable:

- Write short sentences.
- Write short paragraphs (though long enough to cover a particular focus).
- Use simple words.
- Define what you mean, as you go.
- Aim to communicate and not to impress. (1992: 102).

We turn next to some principles concerning the use of specific vocabulary. Hicks states:

> Always write in the third person, not in the first or second person. In other words, use phrases such as 'The subjects were required to …' rather than 'I asked the subjects to …' remember that any research should be objective and disinterested. If you start including 'I', 'me', 'my', 'personally' etc., the report begins to look highly subjective and consequently not very scientific. (1999: 116)

The use of third person is often advocated for reports of quantitative research. It seems to be increasingly acceptable, however, to use the first person in writing up research, rather than the traditional impersonal style. Holloway and Wheeler write:

> The researchers can use the first person, *I*, when they mention what they themselves choose to do. For instance, researchers would not say: the author chose a sample, or the researcher used the methods, etc. They may write: I chose a purposive sample of …, I collected the data through … (1996: 172)

In qualitative research, the use of the first person can be part of recognizing and reflecting on your own role and biases in conducting the research. The danger of using 'I' is the temptation to make unsubstantiated statements of personal belief. It is always best to check the style requirements by asking your supervisor or consulting the 'Information for Authors' if you are writing a paper for a journal.

It is important to be aware of sexism, racism and disablism in your use of language and, indeed, the negative stereotyping of any other group of people. In relation to sexism, you should not attribute characteristics, occupations or exclusively subservient roles to women (for example hysterical woman driver, devoted secretary). The word 'he' should not be used to refer to people in general. The sentence can usually be reworked using a person's name or job/role title (for example the therapist, the client) or using the plural ('they', 'them' etc.).

The following are some specific suggestions. For:

man or mankind – use humanity/human beings/people
girl (for an adult) – use woman
man in the street – use average person
best man for the job – use best person for the job
chairman – use chairperson
spokesman – use spokesperson
saleswoman/salesgirl – use sales representative/sales assistant
manpower – use workforce/staffing

Likewise it is important to avoid racist language and stereotyping people from ethnic minorities. French and Sim state:

> Offensive terms, such as 'coloured' or 'half-caste', though once commonplace in everyday language, are no longer acceptable, and have been replaced by 'black' and 'mixed race'. Even the word 'immigrant' is frequently used in an abusive way. People from these groups are patronizingly overpraised for minor achievements, as if few others like them could achieve so much, and their ethnic origin is frequently referred to unnecessarily as in 'the brilliant black doctor'. (1993: 36)

Stop and Think

Perhaps less recognized is the importance of avoiding dis-ablist language. Along the same lines as the list of sexist lan-guage above, make a list of words and phrases which you feel might be offensive to disabled people and alongside this list make another of more acceptable alternatives.

The following are some suggestions from the British Council of Disabled People: Use the term 'disabled person' rather than the word 'handicapped' or the word 'disabled' as a noun ('the dis-abled'); do not refer to individuals by the medical conditions they have, for instance use 'a person with diabetes' rather than 'a dia-betic'. Avoid some commonly used words; for:

victim – use person who has/with/person who experienced …
crippled by – use person who has/person with …
suffering from – use person who has/person with …
afflicted by – use person who has/person with …
wheelchair bound – use wheelchair user…
mental handicap – use person with learning difficulties …
mental illness – use person with mental health problem/or mental health system survivor …
invalid – use disabled person …

Finally in this section, we turn to strategies to support your writing process. We have already mentioned word-processing. Another important strategy is the use of databases, now most commonly through the use of computer programmes. Databases can be used for the following:

- The storing and retrieving of bibliographical references.
- Storing and retrieving interview data.
- Storing and retrieving numerical data.
- Keeping odd bits of information that are not easily classified.
- Storing ideas for papers, articles, research projects and books.
- Storing quotable quotes.
- Analysing qualitative data.
- Storing and retrieving names and addresses.
- Keeping a track record of a project.
- Collecting and executing 'to-do' lists. (Burnard, 1992: 56)

All of these are useful to do, but we would particularly recommend that first time researchers keep a bibliographical database from the outset. Each card, or 'form' (to use database jargon) should have the following information: the surname of the author followed by the initials; year of publication; title of the book or paper; publisher or name of the journal together with place of publication and journal details (volume, issue, page numbers); keywords; and comments. When you use a direct quotation, keep the page number. Searching for such details later can be frustrating (as we have learnt to our cost).

Structure and contents

The following structure is suitable for most BSc and MSc dissertations as well as research report articles. The structure can be used for PhD theses, though they often follow a different pattern.

Title page
Abstract
Acknowledgements
Table of contents
List of tables and figures
List of appendices
List of abbreviations/Glossary of terms
Introduction
Literature review
Methodology
Results
Discussion
Conclusion
References
Appendices

It is important to recognize that this is only a basic format and many variations are not only possible but desirable. In general terms you should address the audience: who is the report for? And you should gear the report to your particular purposes: what are you seeking to achieve by your report?

There are many possible variations in structure/format of which we shall give just three examples. It is possible to present the findings in the initial chapter. The remainder of the report shows how this conclusion was reached: what was done in the study, how alternative explanations were discarded etc. Second, a narrative report is a straight-forward account of the case study,

essentially told in continuous prose. Third, a chronological structure is basically a format in which the story of the research is
told in chronological sequence.

It is possible to draw out points that are common to *all* report
writing, whether based on a qualitative or quantitative project.
However, it is also important to recognize differences. Basically
there is a conventional format for reporting quantitative research,
while writing up qualitative research can take more varied and
diverse forms. Bannister *et al* advises students writing up qualitative research to, 'be sure that you realize that you are not engaged
in writing up an "experimental report". It is important to ensure
that you are arousing appropriate discourses: avoid using words
such as "experiment", "experimenter", "subject" etc.; instead, talk
about the "researcher", "co-researchers" (or "participants"), etc.'
(1994: 161). We have known students, for instance, use the term
'hypotheses' in reports of qualitative research, and thus make
problems for themselves as their research made no precise predictions which could be subjected to statistical verification.

The first few pages

Title – your title should be informative, specific to your study,
succinct and should engage people's interests. Though you may
well have to provide a possible title in the early stages of
your research, you should not attach too much importance to
this as it will most certainly change as you proceed with your
investigation.

Titles for experimental or quantitative research are perhaps
less creative. Hicks suggests that the title is based on the hypothesis. She gives an example of an experiment with the following
hypothesis: 'Vital capacity is diminished during administration of
lumbar traction for back pain.' Her suggested title is: *An investigation into the relationship between lumbar traction and vital capacity in back pain patients* (1999: 117).

Titles for qualitative research tend to be more difficult to
write as the research itself can be more nebulous and by its
nature 'qualitative'. Silverman suggests a two-part title: a snappy
main title, often using a present participle to indicate activity;
and a subtitle which is descriptive and contains key words

(2000: 222). The following are a couple of examples of chapter titles from a recent research text (Hammell *et al*, 2000):

Working with theory in qualitative research: an example of a study of women with chronic illness (multiple sclerosis);

Understanding another life: using qualitative research in undergraduate education.

You may well find that the title you chose at the start of your research project no longer seems appropriate when you come to write it up. This is because research is a dynamic process which rarely runs entirely smoothly. Some of your original ideas may, for one reason or another, have proved impracticable, and you are likely to have gained new insights as the research progressed, leading to unexpected changes of plan. Whatever the title of your research may be, it should be accurate. Its accuracy will help those who are searching the literature in your particular area to ascertain whether or not your research is relevant to them.

Abstract – the abstract is a précis of your study in just a few hundred words, and although it appears at the beginning of the report it is usually written last. You should state your reasons for doing the research, the methods you used, and your main results and conclusions. It is vital that the abstract is clear, precise and informative. It may be necessary for you to provide a few key words in order for your study to be indexed.

Acknowledgements – you may like to acknowledge those people who have helped you to carry out your project successfully; these may include your tutor, the librarian, the research participants, the funding organization, or a relative or friend. This rarely needs to be more than a paragraph in length and should be placed immediately after the title, or right at the end of the report.

Lists of contents – when you have written the main body of your research report, your final task is to write a list of contents of the various sections, giving the correct page numbers. A list of tables and a list of figures (graphs, diagrams and pictures) should also be included, ensuring that the titles you give tally with the ones in the text. Having read dissertations with distinctly 'user-unfriendly' lists of contents, we would suggest that, though this may seem a trivial task, it is essential in creating 'first impressions'.

Introduction

This needs to begin broadly and progressively focus on, or funnel down to, the particular aims of your study. Start the introduction by giving a broad overall statement describing the general topic and problem being addressed in your research. Then summarize what is known about the problem, that is what others have found out about the problem in their research. Where appropriate summarize different theoretical positions offered to explain the findings of previous research. Finally, identify the gap in the literature that needs to be filled, and then state the purposes of your research. If appropriate, you should state the research hypotheses.

As Holloway and Wheeler (1996) point out, an introduction to a qualitative research study tends to be more personal. It can explain why you have chosen this topic rather than any other, and this can include reasons relating to your professional role and interests.

Literature review

See Chapter 6.

Method or methodology

In reporting quantitative research, this should be structured and concise. This is not a discussion section, but rather a clear description. It is usual to subdivide this section into sub-sections under the following sub-headings:

Design – this covers such things as defining your independent and dependent variables, the sampling design, and the questionnaire design (where relevant to your particular study).

Participants – this sub-section gives all the relevant details about your research participants: age, sex, medical condition, previous treatment etc.

Apparatus – here are the details of any apparatus you used, in sufficient detail so that anyone wanting to replicate the research can obtain the same apparatus.

Materials – this covers details of other materials such as score sheets, assessment techniques, attitude scales and question-naires.

Procedure – here you provide a step-by-step detailed descrip-tion of what you did as you carried out your study in order that others can replicate the study.

Data analysis – it is important to cover the procedures and strategies used for analysing the data, whether the research is qualitative or quantitative.

Ethical issues – ethical issues and how you have dealt with them need to be briefly discussed (see Chapter 3).

The methodology chapter in qualitative research reports can cover ostensibly the same information as above, but as Silverman (2000) argues, the issues covered can differ significantly. One format we have found useful in qualitative research has three sub-headings:

Theoretical assumptions – it is important that this is as concise as possible and links up with discussions in other sections of the report. A summary might be provided, for instance, of the basic methodological assumptions of an interpretive perspective.

Methodological principles – the next step might be to set out some principles in terms of the realization of the theore-tical assumption in research practice. An interpretive perspective can, for instance, underpin a narrative approach (see Chapter 16).

Methodological strategies – Silverman lists the following as important to describe in this sub-section:

- The data you have studied.
- How you obtained those data (for example issues of access and consent).
- What claims you are making about the data (for example as representative of some population or as a single case study).
- The methods you have used to gather the data.
- Why you have chosen these methods.
- How you have analysed your data.
- The advantages and limitations of using your method of data analysis. (2000: 235)

Results

In quantitative research the results chapter is a concise report of the data, often referring to more detailed appendices. Tables or figures can often be used to summarize the data, together with the results of statistical analyses.

The results section should contain the 'facts' of your study. It is usual to begin with the more general results and then move to the more specific findings. If you have a lot of data you may need to be selective in what you present, but you should nonetheless ensure that it provides a well-balanced picture. It is appropriate to give a brief explanation of statistical tests in this section, although detailed statistical information is best placed in an appendix. In order to assist comprehension, you should reduce your raw data to descriptive statistics, tables, graphs, pie charts, etc., making sure that they are labelled accurately and that a key of the symbols you use is provided. The results should be presented in such a way as to make them easy for the reader to assimilate and pleasant to read. Charts and tables should be explained in writing unless their meaning is very obvious. It is important that everything included in this section is there for a purpose. It can be a balancing act between including sufficient information to do justice to your research, but on the other hand not padding out your report with superfluous tables, charts or graphs (no matter how well presented).

When writing up qualitative research, the division between 'results' and 'discussion' is often less distinct. It can be usefully maintained in keeping 'findings' separate from possible 'interpretations'. Although most traditional research texts insist that the results section of research reports should be purely factual and separate from the discussion section, with some qualitative methodologies it is more sensible to combine the two. There are a number of strategies for writing up your data analysis in qualitative research (Silverman, 2000).

1. Make one point at a time
This is not always as easy as it sounds as you should include quotations from participants, and they will not necessarily be making one point at a time. The same quotation can sometimes be used to illustrate more than one point, but the points should be clearly separated.

2. Top and tail each data extract
You need to set each quotation within the general analysis (often referred to as a story) you are developing. Basically, quotations do not speak for themselves.

3. Always show that you understand the limitations of both your data and your analysis of them.
In qualitative research it is always useful to reflect on the research process itself.

4. Be systematic and structured
A qualitative analysis should (usually) be systematic and structured, and your report should reflect this (see Chapter 15).

5. Convince the reader

Silverman writes:

> Not only must your readers be able to see why you interpreted your data in the way you did, they must be convinced by your interpretation. (2000: 246)

Discussion

Jenkins *et al* (1998: 140) recommend that the following should be covered in a discussion of results.

Answer the questions posed in the Introduction
   In quantitative research, you should return first to the hypotheses. What are the findings of the study in relation to the predictions made by the hypotheses?
Explain the findings
Compare the findings with other research on the topic
Discuss the limitations of the findings
Discuss the implications of the findings and recommend changes for professional practice
Make recommendations for further research (though this might be included in the Conclusion).
   It is particularly important to make clear the limitations of your study in this section, as well as pointing out any major problems you encountered. Your sample may, for example, have been insufficiently large to allow generalizations of your findings to be made; the return rate of your questionnaire study may have been low; and a key person may have withdrawn at the last minute. It is important to reflect on the ethical issues you encountered in the process of research. If you are writing the research project as part of your course work, mistakes and shortcomings are unlikely to have an adverse affect upon your grade, provided you own up to them. Indeed, developing your understanding of research processes is likely to be an explicit aim of any research project which is part of course work and critical reflection on how you conducted the research will be expected and encouraged.

Conclusion

The conclusion can be written as a separate section or as a paragraph or two at the end of the discussion. It is important that any conclusions you draw really do result from your study, rather than from the work of others or what you hoped your study would reveal. The conclusion should highlight the main points of your research and emphasize those issues and controversies which you hope the reader will remember. It is usual again to reflect critically on the whole research process and to suggest possibilities for further research.

References

All the references you used in your study must be written in full so that interested persons can locate them without difficulty. There are many referencing systems from which to choose, but whichever one you use it is important to be consistent. With the Harvard system the names of authors with the dates are written in the text, with all the references listed alphabetically at the end of the study. Alternatively with the Vancouver system each reference is given a small number in the text and the references are listed at the end in the order of these numbers. You may also like to list the books and articles you found helpful in conducting your research, but which do not appear in your text. This listing can be headed 'Bibliography' and placed after your list of references. (For full details of various systems of referencing, you are referred to French and Sim, 1993.)

Appendices

Detailed information which would interfere with the flow of your text, or which only the more meticulous readers would wish to consult, should be located in the appendices which are placed at the end of your report. Even here it is important to be selective. Items suitable for inclusion include questionnaires, interview and observation schedules, raw data, letters, details of apparatus, details of statistical tests, and lists of organizations. You need to be careful not to inadvertently break confidentiality, for instance by including a hospital address or a participant's signature.

Conclusion

It is important to emphasize again that 'writing up' is a form of communication. In reports of quantitative research, there tends to be a much more set format, but most marks are usually gained through the quality of the discussion sections. It is essential that the report reads as an organic whole, rather than as a set of separate independent sections. In working out your timescale for a project you should leave yourself time to read and edit the document as a whole.

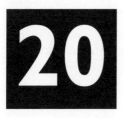

Making public: Dissemination

How, why and to whom?

It can be argued that 'making public' is part of the definition of 'research'. An activity can have all the usual characteristics of research, data collection and analysis etc., but remains in the realms of personal and professional development until it is made public.

Stop and Think

You have been involved, as a member of a multidisciplinary team, investigating the provision of therapy for physically disabled pupils in two schools which have a policy of inclusion. This involved interviewing disabled pupils, their parents, teachers and other professionals to explore the views and experiences of the provision of therapy within the two schools. The research team has analysed the data and the project has, you feel, been successful in terms of producing some interesting findings.

So what next? You've reached the stage of making the findings public. List six possible ways of disseminating your findings.

There are numerous possibilities which can be thought of in terms of types or modes of communication.

1. Written presentation

The most obvious are written reports of research findings. There are a wide variety of possibilities here, including academic journal papers, professional journals or newsletters, research project reports, booklets, and book chapters.

2. Verbal presentation

This could be through a presentation at a conference, sessions for students or staff training, departmental seminars and special interest group meetings (recognizing of course that such presentations are not solely verbal).

3. Media presentation

Here we could include video or audio presentation. The fastest growing way of presenting research findings in the past ten years has to be through the Internet. There are, of course, the public media of television, radio and newspapers.

There are various ways of disseminating research findings and the means selected by therapists is a question in itself. Jenkins *et al* reflect a widely accepted belief.

> Journal articles are the most effective and permanent means of disseminating information to a large audience. (1998: 94)

Many researchers, however, disseminate their research in different ways to different audiences. It is quite possible to disseminate the same research project through a presentation at a conference, a paper in a professional journal, a paper in an academic journal, and on the Internet, as well as summative reports for those directly involved in the project.

Before looking at some of these methods in more detail, we need to consider another general question, that is the purposes of dissemination. It is not just a matter of communicating findings. There are at least four main reasons for disseminating research: to inform others of the findings; to try to ensure that the research is used; to meet obligations to participants; and to clarify interpretations and recommendations. As Fuller and Petch (1995) suggest, the findings and recommendations may be challenging to existing therapy practice, to the assumptions on which practice is based, and to organizational vested interests. If you wish your research to make an impact, it is likely that you will have to work for this. Furthermore, dissemination may not take place only after the completion of the research. There can be good reasons for aiming at rapid or interim feedback. It can be part of your obligations as a researcher to disseminate findings to participants before disseminating to a wider audience. In more participatory approaches this can be part of the research process, seeking respondent validation and promoting further discussion.

Stop and Think
The third way of considering dissemination is the question, to whom? Who is the target audience? Return to the *Stop and Think* activity above. To which groups might the modes of communication be directed? List three possible audiences for the findings for this research project.

It is important to tailor the communication of your findings to the particular audience you are addressing. There are a number of categories, or groups, to which the findings can be communicated.

1. Research participants
The first audience has to be those directly involved in the research. In this research there are three groups of participants: pupils, parents and professionals. It can also include any funders of the research.

2. The professional or practitioner audience
The second most obvious audience is fellow professionals. The findings of participants' views and experiences in the two schools will be of interest to a wider audience of professionals involved with the inclusion of disabled pupils in educational settings.

3. The policy-making audience

4. The lay audience

5. The academic audience

Publishing

An important way of disseminating your research findings is to publish them in relevant journals and newspapers. The format for presenting your research will be similar to that of the research report, but the material will need to be far more condensed. This can be difficult when you have written a 100,000 word thesis. With larger scale research projects it can be helpful to think in terms of several papers with different foci. Certainly deciding on the storyline (or focus) can be a crucial point in writing a paper. Remember that journal editors work about three months in advance and sometimes a lot longer, so if you want your article to be published by a specific date it should be sent in good time.

Before presenting either your ideas or your work to a journal editor, it is essential that you carry out some thorough market research. You should write your article with a particular journal in mind and only present your ideas to an editor who is likely to be interested in them. Some research projects can be disseminated through different journal outlets, for instance within both an academic and a professional journal. Have a really good look at likely journals and magazines to see if your work is appropriate. Note the length and content of articles, the length of sentences and paragraphs, and the complexity of the language. It is vital to bear the readership in mind when deciding what to present and how to structure your article; a general readership would, for example, require a rather different approach to a readership of therapists.

It is important too to look at the *Information for authors* usually found on the inside of the front or back cover of journals. The journal *Physiotherapy* is a typical example. The information for authors begins with a statement about the journal, what the editors are wanting to achieve. It then provides lists of the types of articles it publishes. It also provides details about such things as: the preparation of material for presentation to the editors (line spacing etc.), including the referencing style; copyright; permissions and ethical certification; and submission of articles. When you have decided which journal to approach, it can help to talk to the editor about your ideas before proceeding to write, as a similar article may already have been accepted.

In the case of professional journals, your article will go through a peer review system where its suitability for publication will be judged. More often than not you will be asked to make modifications and amendments. Usually the request to make changes will be accompanied by comments and suggestions from two anonymous referees and responding to these is something of an art in itself. Some comments can be very specific, such as suggested literature not referred to in the article, or quite general, for example that the literature review in the article is weak (without specific suggestions being given). We have found that the two referees quite often make very different suggestions, and occasionally found the reviews contradict each other (one being totally positive while the other is damning). We have found the following to be generally useful strategies in redrafting papers.

- It is a good strategy to list the referees' suggestions and make a few notes summarizing changes you have made to the paper in response to each suggestion, with cross-references to the relevant pages and paragraphs in the revised manuscript.
- As far as possible respond positively to their recommendations. Many involve small changes, even corrections of grammatical and spelling errors.
- Sometimes it is possible to edit out rather than revise a short section, sentence or paragraph, that a referee has found problematic. Often these are points which diverge from the main argument or analysis.
- Sometimes when a referee has disagreed with a point being made it is possible to strengthen or justify your original argument rather than following the referee's recommendation. It is a good idea to explicitly defend your approach in the covering letter, if you disagree with a reviewer's sugges-

tions, to show the editor that you have considered the suggestion carefully.

● If your manuscript is rejected try not to throw it in the bin (though this can be a natural response). It may be that you sent it to an inappropriate journal.

It is our experience that redrafting a paper in response to referees' comments almost invariably improves it. Also, with professional and academic journals, page proofs are supplied for authors to correct before the article is published; changes to the article will not be made without the author's permission.

With the more light-weight newspapers, the editor will normally decide whether or not to publish your work. If it is accepted you will be informed and it will appear in the newspaper a few weeks or months later. You will not normally receive proofs to correct and your article may be changed by the editorial staff without your permission. In this way research results are sometimes distorted or the general 'tone' of the article is changed, for instance by the adoption of an inappropriate, ostensibly more catchy, title or illustration.

Despite the possible distortion of your research findings when submitting them to the popular press, in many ways this is a more satisfactory way of disseminating research data, inasmuch as more people tend to read popular newspapers and magazines than prestigious, academic journals. Writing for the popular press is, however, rarely encouraged in academic and professional circles.

Presentations

Verbal presentations

Verbal presentations are a crucial vehicle for disseminating research ideas and findings. This includes the presentation of a paper at scientific or professional conferences, conducting a research seminar at a university or hospital department, and presenting research as part of academic studies. The last of these would include an oral examination for a PhD. There are many positive reasons for undertaking a verbal presentation. Once you have gone to the work of condensing your findings for a presentation, it may be easier to turn the material into a journal article, as the 'storyline' will have become much clearer.

Stop and Think

A good starting point for thinking about verbal presentations is your own experiences as a member of the audience at a conference, seminar or a lecture. What makes a good presentation? Make a list of what you think are the main five characteristics of a good oral presentation. (Memories of what you felt were poor presentations can be helpful in this.)

From our experiences we would suggest the following:

● The presentation is tailored to the specific audience.
● The presenter 'engages' with the audience.
● The focus is quite narrow and the presenter does not ramble around a number of disparate issues.
● The presentation is varied with good use of audiovisual aids and illustrative practical or specific examples.
● The content of the presentation is well structured with emphasis being given to the main points being made.

Giving a talk about your research will come at the end of a much longer process of planning it; you should aim to make your talk interesting, stimulating and coherent. A verbal presentation of research normally includes a brief introduction, a statement of purpose, an account of methodology and procedure, a consideration of the major findings, and the researcher's own conclusions and recommendations.

If you decide to disseminate your research findings by means of a talk, careful consideration must be given both to its content and your presentation. When offering a presentation to a conference, you will need to send an abstract, which itself is well focused, interesting and, where necessary, engages with the conference theme. The most important thing to remember in a presentation is the audience: What is their particular interest in your research? What is the state of their knowledge on the topic? How does your research apply to their situation? Your talk will obviously be more difficult to prepare and present if people in the audience have different levels of knowledge, with some knowing nothing about the topic and others knowing more than you do.

It is not usually satisfactory to read aloud from detailed notes when giving a talk. Reading verbatim from notes tends to sound dry and dull, and has the effect of distancing the speaker from the audience. It is best to talk in a clear, conversational style, keeping engaged with the audience, and avoiding jargon and unnecessary detail. If you have had little or no experience of giving talks, you may, understandably, find the prospect of doing so without a detailed record rather alarming, but your performance will almost certainly benefit if you are sufficiently familiar with what you need to say to manage with the use of cards containing a few 'trigger' words or phrases. You can always keep your detailed notes close at hand for reassurance or emergency.

It is likely that your talk will be constrained within a strict time limit. This means that you will need to be very selective with regard to what you present, perhaps restricting yourself to one particular theme of your research. The most common mistake when giving a talk is to cram too much in; it is best to concentrate on the major themes rather than the detail. If you want to give more detailed information you can provide your audience with a handout or a reference list to follow up. It is best, when giving a talk, to speak a little slower than normal; verbalizing the talk to yourself, or recording it and playing it back, will help you judge the timing as well as building your confidence.

Whatever the length of your talk, it is vital that you hold the attention of your audience; the longer your presentation the more difficult this will be. One way of enhancing attention is to use a variety of audio-visual aids, for example slides, video and the overhead projector. All visual aids should be clear, simple, uncluttered and relevant, with an accurate match between their content and what is being said (French *et al*, 1994). Perhaps the most commonly used visual aid is the overhead projector. This is a way of presenting the main points of the presentation or diagrams. A more recent innovation which has opened up many different possibilities for enhancing verbal presentations is through the use of computers, and in particular *Powerpoint*. It is also important that the needs of disabled members of the audience are taken into consideration, for example those with hearing or visual impairments (London Borough's Disability Resource Team, 1991).

Another way of holding the attention of your audience, and increasing their enjoyment and satisfaction, is to encourage them to express their views and ask questions. Throwing the floor open to questions and possible criticism takes courage; a way of reducing the anxiety of this is to present your talk to some supportive but critical colleagues as a means of rehearsal. A further advantage of this is that it will provide you with feedback on your presentation and will help you to verify the timing of your talk.

To reduce unnecessary worry just before giving a talk, you should check all the equipment you intend to use and familiarize yourself with the room; if your talk is part of a conference it can be very reassuring to listen to an earlier speaker. Once you have started the talk, focusing your attention on the needs of the audience rather than on yourself can help to reduce anxiety. Be sensitive to their non-verbal communication, and make sure they can see the visual displays you present and hear you clearly. Do not be unduly concerned or embarrassed if you cannot answer every question you are asked, or if you agree with some of the criticisms made of your research. Never try to cover up errors or gaps in your knowledge; audiences usually respect honest, open speakers. As the presenter you are responsible for the overall mood of the group; a little humour can help you gain rapport with your audience, but only if it comes naturally to you. Some degree of anxiety is not a bad thing as it will stimulate you to give your best.

The oral examination or 'viva' associated with PhD research is a very specific type of verbal presentation, for very specific purposes. The 'viva' is conducted by external and internal examiners whose task it is to establish whether you have demonstrated that you are a 'fully professional researcher who should be listened to because you can make a sensible contribution to the development of your field' (Phillips and Pugh, 1994: 139). Silverman (2000: 258) provides a list of suggestions for preparing for an oral examination:

- Revise your thesis.
- Prepare a list of points you want to get across.
- Find out about your external/internal examiners' work.
- Practise with others in a mock viva.

He also provides a list of 'tips for the oral examination', adapted below, which can be seen as having a general application.

- Always say if you have not understood a question; if so, ask for more clarification.
- Use the questions as opportunities to get your point across by making links between the questions and the things you want to say. Though make sure that you do address the questions.
- Avoid overlong answers which drift very far from the original question.
- Refer to the list of points you want to get across when your examiners ask whether there is anything they have not covered.
- Ask your supervisor to make notes of questions and answers. The discussion in verbal presentations generally can be of use to you in revising your thesis or preparing a paper for publication.

Poster presentations

Poster presentations are a mode of summarizing and communicating research in a primarily visual format. Posters should be concise, eye-catching, appealing, informative and interactive with the viewers. As Wilson and Hutchinson point out, this can be relatively easy when reporting quantitative findings in colourful pie charts and bar graphs, but more challenging in qualitative research when findings consist of 'stories concepts, description, explanation, and grounded theories' (1997: 68).

Poster presentations can be particularly useful at an early stage in the research dissemination. They can provide feedback for you by stimulating discussions with audiences who are pursuing research into the same or similar topics or are familiar with the methodological issues you are raising. Many conferences include formal poster sessions where presenters are expected to be available for discussion. If there are no such sessions, you can be available during key viewing times, such as during lunch breaks. The possibility for in-depth discussions with interested people can make poster presentations particularly useful.

Wilson and Hutchinson (1997: 70–80) provide a useful breakdown of concerns in preparing a poster presentation which we have adapted below.

Targeting your audience
The choice of one meeting or conference over another requires that you identify the audience you wish to interact with in presenting a summary of your research, often research in-progress, for example researchers, professionals, or both.

Obtaining official guidelines
It is important to obtain guidelines from the conference or meeting organizers as to the dimensions and type of expected poster displays.

Designing a poster presentation
Space is obviously at a premium when designing a poster. It must look striking and interesting and be easy to read. The lettering should be more than 5 mm in height, and the text should be broken up with diagrams, photographs, graphs or pictures as appropriate. The use of colour can serve to enliven the poster. Desktop publishing software can be invaluable when constructing the poster, as can the help and advice of a graphic artist. Some poster displays also make use of other audio and visual exhibits which are relevant to the research, such as a short video, a tape recording, or an explanatory model. A handout or a list of references can also be provided.

Morra (1984) (in Wilson and Hutchinson, 1997) provides a set of principles for poster presentations that include the following:

- Less is better. Don't try to say too much.
- Bigger is better. Don't crowd your exhibit.
- Write headlines (panel titles) with brief, colourful nouns and vigorous active verbs.
- Five times as many viewers read headlines as read text copy.
- Headlines that promise the reader a benefit, contain news or offer helpful information attract above average readership.
- There is evidence too that people find it harder to read capitals, so posters need to avoid placing headings and subheadings solely in capital letters.
- Help your readers with arrows, bullets or other mark.
- Use subheadings every two to three inches.
- Photos are better than drawings.
- Write a caption for every graph or illustration. People read text under illustrations. We would add that you will need to give thought to the accessibility of your presentation. Large print handouts, for instance, should be available for people with visual impairments.

The content
What you display will depend on your particular research topic, but as Jenkins et al (1998) suggest, it will usually include seven main sections: the title of your project; authors' names, titles and designations; introduction including the main reason for carrying it out; a brief description of the methods you used; often most importantly, your major results (when appropriate in graphic or tabular form); and your conclusions, including recommendations.

The construction
Desktop publishing software has found increasing use in generating posters. These programmes provide for flexibility in placing text and graphics. Each of the panels can be headed with an institution logo. Consideration needs to be given too to the

materials used for your research poster, remembering any possible difficulties in transportation.

Ethical issues

Ethical dilemmas are no less prevalent at the stage of reporting and disseminating research findings than throughout the research process. As Seale and Barnard recognize, 'ethical issues in dissemination include the areas of anonymity, confidentiality, copyright and accuracy of reporting' (1998: 228). As to the last of these, omitting information, falsifying data, and outright fraud among both professional researchers and students, usually caused by pressures to succeed, are well documented in the literature. Selection of data to include in a report and the interpretation of findings can raise ethical issues. Glass argues that researchers have a responsibility to report the results of clinical trials accurately, including 'complete and accurate reporting of efficacy criteria, side effects, editorial decisions not to report negative findings' (1994: 336). Failure to report accurately may result in harm to clients.

Researchers may choose to omit findings in order to protect participants or themselves, and knowledge is selected and shaped by editors and the peer review system. It is far more difficult, for example, to get research which is not statistically significant published, than that which is, leading to bias and distortion in the knowledge produced. Publishers operate with a view to the market, which can prevent the publication of certain types of knowledge while shaping and structuring that which is produced. When research is disseminated, researchers tend to lose control of it, and it may be used in ways of which they disapprove.

Ideally, research findings should be made available to the public and research participants, but whether or not they are depends, to a large extent, on how they are disseminated. The right to publish may be limited by sponsors, and career advancement may induce researchers to place their work in prestigious journals which few people read.

The publication of qualitative research can carry the risks and potential harm from identification of informants, individuals, an institution and/or a group. The recognition of participants in print can have harmful consequences: damage to reputations, interference with personal or family relationships, and some-times endangerment (Lipson, 1997). Publication may also lead to feelings of betrayal or embarrassment through participants seeing things in print they may have said very casually. Damage to reputation and endangerment can result from the publication of participants' involvement in potentially stigmatizing or illegal activities or situations (past or present). Lipson (1997: 47) pro-vides a comprehensive list of strategies or techniques to protect participants. These include:

- Delay publication.
- Seek the approval of participants before publication.
- Omit potentially damaging details.
- Use pseudonyms or code numbers.
- Remove identifying material from transcripts.
- Change demographic data not central to 'the story'.

Finally, Sapsford and Abbott state: 'another problem is the use to which our research findings are put – often completely unintended by the researchers themselves. Findings may be interpreted in ways that are much to the disadvantage of the researched' (1996: 322). The example they give is research meant to demonstrate the hardships of those experiencing poverty which was interpreted as demonstrating that the problem was the way income was spent. As emphasized earlier, dissemination can be something that you need to work at and researchers cannot absolve themselves from the uses made of their research.

Conclusion: Disseminate and be damned

The phrase, of course, is 'publish and be damned', and we have just broadened it. As evident ftom the above discussion, however, we do not mean be damned by contravening ethical principles. Three general aims in therapist research are: staff/therapist development, improvement of therapy practice, and the development and construction of theories of therapy. The achievement of these aims is simply not possible without at least some dissemination of the research. Research has a role to play in promoting change and, though dissemination cannot guarantee change, 'dissemination is still one vital component of the process and should be undertaken' (Bowling, 1997: 141).

References

Alasuutari, P. (1995) *Researching Culture: Qualitative method and cultural studies*, Sage, London

Annual Report (1959–60) *Barclay School for Partially Sighted Girls*

Argyrous, G. (2000) *Statistics for Social and Health Research*, Sage, London

Arksey, A. and Knight, P. (1999) *Interviewing for Social Scientists*, Sage, London

Armitstead, J. (1997) An Evaluation of Initial Non-Attendance Rates for Physiotherapy. *Physiotherapy*, **83(11)**, 591–596

Atkinson, D. (1993a) Relating. In Shakespeare, P., Atkinson, D. and French, S. (eds) *Reflecting on Research Practice: Issues in health and social welfare*, Open University Press, Buckingham

Atkinson, D. (ed) (1993b) *Past Times: Older people with learning difficulties look back on their lives*, Open University Press, Buckingham

Atkinson, D. (1999) An old story. In Swain, J. and French, S. (eds) *Therapy and Learning Difficulties: Advocacy, participation and partnership*, Butterworth-Heinemann, Oxford

Atkinson, D., Jackson, M. and Walmsley, J. (1997) *Forgotten Lives: Exploring the history of learning disability*, British Institute of Learning Disabilities, Kidderminster

Babbie, E. (1992) *The Practice of Social Research* (6th ed.), Wadsworth Publishing, Belmont, California

Bailey, D. M. (1991) *Research for the Health Professions*, F. A. Davis, Philadelphia

Banister, P., Burman, E., Parker, I., Taylor, M. and Tindall, C. (1996)

Qualitative Research in Psychology: A research guide, Open University Press, Buckingham

Barclay, J. (1999) A Historical Review of Learning Difficulties, Remedial Therapy and the Rise of the Professional Therapist. In Swain, J. and French, S. (eds) *Therapy and Learning Difficulties: Advocacy, participation and partnership*, Butterworth-Heinemann, Oxford

Barnard, S. (1995) Wessex Region Physiotherapy Audit Project: Models for intervention audit, *Physiotherapy*, **81(4)**, 202–207

Barnard, S. and Hartigan, G. (1998) *Clinical Audit in Physiotherapy: From theory into practice*, Butterworth-Heinemann, Oxford

Barnes, C. (1992) Qualitative Research: Valuable or irrelevant? *Disability, Handicap and Society*, **7(2)**,115–124

Barton, L. (1998) Developing an Emancipatory Research Agenda: Possibilities and dilemmas. In Clough, P. and Barton, L. (eds) *Articulating with Difficulty: Research voices in inclusive education*, Paul Chapman, London

Beeston, S., Rastall, M. and Hoare, C. (1998) Factors Influencing the Uptake of Taught Master's Programmes Among Physiotherapists. *Physiotherapy*, **84(10)**, 480–486

Bell, J. (1999) *Doing Your Research Project: A guide for first-time researchers in education and social science* (3rd ed.), Open University Press, Buckingham

Beratta, R. (1996) A Critical Review of the Delphi Technique. *Nurse Researcher*, **3(4)**, 59–69

Biggerstaff, D., Macarthur, C., Bick, D. *et al* (2000) Postnatal Care – Women's Help-Seeking Behaviour and Their Views about Health. *Journal of Reproductive and Infant Psychology*, **18(3)**, 255

Bines, H., Swain, J. and Kaye, J. (1998) 'Once upon a time': Teamwork for complementary perspectives and critique in research on special educational needs. In Clough, P. and Barton, L. (eds) *Articulating with Difficulty: Research voices in inclusive education*, Paul Chapman, London

Birkett, M. (1995) Is Audit Action Research? *Physiotherapy*, **81(4)**, 190–194

Blanche, E. I. (1996) Alma: Coping with culture, poverty, and disability. *The American Journal of Occupational Therapy*, **50(4)**, 265–276

Bornat, J. (1993) Presenting. In Shakespeare, P., Atkinson, D. and

French, S. (eds) *Reflecting on Research Practice: Issues in health and social welfare*, Open University Press, Buckingham

Bowling, A. (1997) *Research Methods in Health: Investigating health and health services*, Open University Press, Buckingham

Boyd Boonyawiroj, E. (1996) Physiotherapy Re-entry: A case study. *Physiotherapy*, **82(8)**, 447–455

Braye, S. (2000) Participation and Involvement in Social Care: An overview. In Kemshall, H. and Littlechild, R. (eds) *User Involvement and Participation in Social Care: Research informing practice*, Jessica Kingsley, London

Brechin, A. (1993) Sharing. In Shakespeare, P., Atkinson, D. and French, S. (eds) *Reflecting on Research Practice: Issues in health and social welfare*, Open University Press, Buckingham

Britton, C. (1999) A Pilot Study Exploring Families' Experience of Caring for Children with Chronic Arthritis: Views from the inside. *British Journal of Occupational Therapy*, **62(12)**, 534–542

Brown, R. (1988) *Group Processes*, Blackwell, Oxford

Bryman, A. (1988) *Quantity and Quality in Social Research*, Unwin Hyman, London

Burnard, P. (1992) *Writing for Health Professionals: A manual for writers*, Chapman and Hall, London

Burr, V. (1995) *An Introduction to Social Constructionism*, Routledge, London

Carpenter, C. and Hammell, K. (2000) Evaluating Qualitative Research. In Hammell, K. W., Carpenter, C. and Dyck, I. (eds) *Using Qualitative Research: A practical introduction for occupational and physical therapists*, Churchill Livingstone, Edinburgh

Chalmers, I. and Altman, D. (1995) *Systematic Reviews*, BMJ Publishing Group, London

Chambers, R. (1997) *Whose Reality Counts: Putting the first last*, Intermediate Technology Publications, London

College of Occupational Therapists (1998) *Clinical Audit Information Pack: A resource pack to assist occupational therapists with clinical audit and clinical effectiveness*, College of Occupational Therapy, London

Coolidge, F. (2000) *Statistics: A gentle introduction*, London, Sage

Cornwall, A. and Jewkes, R. (1995) What is Participatory Research? *Social Science and Medicine*, **41(12)**, 1667–1676

Costley, D. (2000) Collecting the Views of Young People with

Moderate Learning Difficulties. In Lewis, A. and Lindsey, G. (eds) *Researching Children's Perspectives*, Open University Press, Buckingham

COT (1995) *Code of Ethics and Professional Conduct for Occupational Therapists*, College of Occupational Therapists, London

Crocker, M., MacKay-Lyons, M. and McDonnell, E. (1997) Forced Use of the Upper Extremity in Cerebral Palsy: A single-case design. *American Journal of Occupational Therapy*, **51(10)**, 824–833

Cross, V. (1999) The Same but Different: A Delphi study of clinicians' and academics' perceptions of physiotherapy undergraduates *Physiotherapy*, **85(1)**, 28–39

CSP (1996) *Rules of Professional Conduct*, Chartered Society of Physiotherapy, London

CST (1988) *Code of Ethics and Professional Conduct, with Ethical Guidelines for Research*, College of Speech Therapists, London

de Koning, K. and Martin, M. (1996) Participatory Research in Health: Setting the context. In de Koning, K. and Martin, M. (eds) *Participatory Research in Health: Issues and experiences*, Zed Books, London

Denscombe, M. (1998) *The Good Research Guide: For small-scale social research projects*, Open University Press, Buckingham,

Denzin, N. K. (1989) *Interpretive Biography*, Sage, London

Diamantopoulos, A. and Schlegelmich, B. (1997) *Taking the Fear Out of Data Analysis*, Dryden Press, London

Dobson, C. (1995) Record Audit: A study of the quality and effectiveness of the treatment of knee conditions. *Physiotherapy*, **81(4)**, 218–221

Domholdt, E. (2000) *Physical Therapy Research: Principles and applications* (2nd ed.), W. B. Saunders Company, Philadelphia

Donabedian, A. (1992) Quality Assurance: Structure, process and outcome (interview). *Nursing Standard*, **7(11 Suppl. QA)**, 4–5

Eames, J, Ward, G. and Siddons, L. (1999) Clinical Audit of the Outcome of Individualised Occupational Therapy Goals. *British Journal of Occupational Therapy*, **62(6)**, 257–260

English National Board for Nursing (1998) Research: Getting it funded. *Nursing Standard*, **12(25)**, 11–17

Erlandson, D. A., Harris, E. L., Skipper, B. L. and Allen, S. D. (1993) *Doing Naturalistic Inquiry: A guide to methods*, Sage, Newbury Park

Finnegan, R. (1996) Using Documents. In Sapsford, R. and Jupp, V. (eds) *Data Collection and Analysis*, Sage, London

Fook, J. (ed) (1996) *The Reflective Researcher*, Allen and Unwin, London

Foster, S. B. (1987) *The Politics of Caring*, Falmer Press, London

Foster, P. (1996) Observational Research. In Sapsford, R. and Jupp, V. (eds) *Data Collection and Analysis*, Sage, London

Frank, G. (1996) Life Histories in Occupational Therapy Clinical Practice. *The American Journal of Occupational Therapy*, **50(4)**, 251–264

French, S. (1993) Telling. In Shakespeare, P., Atkinson, D. and French, S. (eds) *Reflecting on Research Practice: Issues in health and social welfare*, Open University Press, Buckingham

French, S. (1996) Out of Sight Out of Mind: The experience and effects of a 'special' residential school. In Morris, J. (ed) *Encounters with Strangers: Feminism and disability*, The Women's Press, London

French, S. (1997) Why Do People Become Patients? In French, S. (ed) *Physiotherapy: A psychosocial approach* (2nd ed.), Butterworth-Heinemann, Oxford

French, S. (1999) Multidisciplinary teams. In Swain, J. and French, S. (eds) *Therapy and Learning Difficulties: Advocacy, participation and partnership*, Butterworth-Heinemann, Oxford

French, S. (2000) *Barriers and Coping Strategies: A study of the working lives of visually impaired physiotherapists*, Unpublished PhD Thesis, Open University

French, S. and Sim, J. (1993) *Writing: A guide for therapists*, Butterworth-Heinemann, Oxford

French, S., Neville, S. and Laing, J. (1994) *Teaching and Learning: A guide for therapists*, Butterworth-Heinemann, Oxford

Fuller, D. and Petch, A. (1995) *Practitioner Research: The reflexive social worker*, Open University Press, Buckingham

Gates, M. F. and Lackey, N. R. (2000) The Researcher Experience in Health Care Research with Families. In Moch, S. D. and Gates, M. F. (eds) *The Researcher Experience in Qualitative Research*, Sage, Thousand Oaks

Gilkeson, G. E. (1997) *Occupational Therapy Leadership: Marketing yourself, your profession and your organization*, F. A. Davis Company, Philadelphia

Gillman, M. (1999) Reflective Practice and Practitioner Research. In Swain, J. and French, S. (eds) (1999) *Therapy and Learning Difficulties: Advocacy, participation and partnership*, Butterworth-Heinemann, Oxford

Gillman, M., Swain, J. and Heyman, B. (1997) Life History or 'Case' History: The objectification of people with learning difficulties through the tyranny of professional discourses. *Disability and Society*, **12(5)**, 675–693

Glass, K. C. (1996) Towards a Duty to Report Clinical Trials Accurately: The clinical alert and beyond. *The Journal of Law, Medicine and Ethics*, **22**, 327–338

Glastonbury, B. and MacKean, J. (1991) Survey Methods. In Allan, G. and Skinner, S. (eds) *A Handbook for Students in the Social Sciences*, Falmer Press, London

Glickman, S. and Kamm, M. (1996) Bowel Dysfunction in Spinal-Cord-Injury Patients. *Lancet*, **347(9016)**, 1651–1653, June 15

Goffman, E. (1961) *Asylums*, Penguin Books, Harmondsworth

Goodley, D. (1996) Tales of Hidden Lives: A critical examination of life history research with people who have learning difficulties. *Disability and Society*, **11(3)**, 333–348

Graham, P., Jordan, A. and Lamb, B. (1990) *An Equal Chance or No Chance?* The Spastics Society, London

Green, S. (1996) Travelling via Delphi: A new route to the accreditation of fieldwork educators. *British Journal of Occupational Therapy*, **59(11)** 506–510

Green, A. (1997) An Audit of Occupational Therapy Outpatient Attendance. *British Journal of Occupational Therapy*, **60(9)**, 384–388

Hammell, K. W. (2000) Representation and Accountability in Qualitative Research. In Hammell, K. W., Carpenter, C. and Dyck, I. (2000) *Using Qualitative Research: A practical introduction for occupational and physical therapists*, Churchill Livingstone, Edinburgh

Hammell, K. W., Carpenter, C. and Dyck, I. (2000) *Using Qualitative Research: A practical introduction for occupational and physical therapists*, Churchill Livingstone, Edinburgh

Hammerskey, M. and Atkinson, P. (1983) *Ethnography: Principles in practice*, Tavistock Publications, London

Haralambos, M. and Holborn, M. (1990) *Sociology: Themes and perspectives* (3rd ed.), Collins Educational, London

Hart, E. and Bond, M. (1995) *Action Research for Health and Social Care: A guide to practice*, Open University Press, Buckingham

Haworth, G. (1993) *Ethical Issues in Student Research in Occupational Therapy: Some guidelines for good practice*, Canterbury Christ Church College, Canterbury

Heck, S. (1989) The Effect of Purposeful Activity on Pain Tolerance. *American Journal of Occupational Therapy*, **42(9)**, 577–581

Heyman, B., Swain, J., Gillman, M., Handyside, E. C. and Newman, W. (1997) Alone in the Crowd: How adults with learning difficulties cope with social network problems. *Social Science and Medicine*, **44**, 41–53

Hick, C. M. (1999) *Research Methods for Clinical Therapists: Applied project design and analysis* (3rd ed.), Churchill Livingstone, Edinburgh

Hilton, R. W. (1995) Fragmentation Within Interprofessional Work: A result of isolationism in health care professional education programmes and the preparation of students to function only in the confines of their own disciplines. *Journal of Interprofessional Care*, **9(1)**, 33–40

Hirsch, K. (1995) Culture and Disability: The role of oral history. *Oral History Review*, **22(1)**, 1–27

Hitch, P. J. and Murgatroyd, J. D. (1983) Professional Communication and Cancer Care: A Delphi study of hospital nurses. *Journal of Advanced Nursing*, **8**, 413–422

Holloway, I. and Wheeler, S. (1996) *Qualitative Research for Nurses*, Blackwell Science, Oxford

Hollway, W. and Jefferson, T. (2000) *Doing Qualitative Research Differently: Free association, narrative and the interview methods*, Sage, London

Holmes, B. and Johnson, A. (1988) *Cold Comfort*, Souvenir Press, London

Homan, R. (1991) *The Ethics of Social Research*, Longman, Harlow

Hsieh, C., Nelson, D., Smith, D. and Peterson, C. (1996) A Comparison of Performance in Added-Purpose Occupations and Rote Exercise for Dynamic Standing Balance in Persons with Hemiplegia. *American Journal of Occupational Therapy*, **50(1)**,10–16

Jenkins, S., Price, C. J. and Straker, L. (1998) *The Researching Therapist: A practical guide to planning, performing and communicating research*, Churchill Livingstone, Edinburgh

Jepson, J. (1998) Study into the Equipment Needs of People with Restrictive Growth. *British Journal of Occupational Therapy*, **61(1)**, 22–26

Johnson, C. and Sim, J. (1998) AIDS and HIV: A comparative study of therapy students' knowledge and attitudes. *Physiotherapy*, **84(1)**, 37–46

Jones, C. and Tannock J. (2000) A Matter of Life and Death: A reflective account of two examples of practitioner research into children's understanding and experience of death and bereavement. In Lewis, A. and Lindsey, G. (eds) *Researching Children's Perspectives*, Open University Press, Buckingham

Jordan, K., Ong, B. and Croft, P. (1998) *Mastering Statistics: A guide for health service professionals and researchers*, Stanley Thornes, Cheltenham

Judd, C., Smith, E. R. and Kidder, L. H. (1991) *Research Methods in Social Relations* (6th ed.), Holt, Rinehart and Winston, London

Kamwendo, K., Askenbom, M. and Wahlgren, C. (1999) Physical Activity in the Life of the Patient with Rheumatoid Arthritis. *Physiotherapy Research International*, **4(4)**, 278–292

Kemmis, S. and McTaggart, R. (2000) Participatory Action Research. In Denzin, N. K. and Lincoln, Y. S. (eds) *Handbook of Qualitative Research* (2nd ed.), Sage, Thousand Oaks

Kemshall, H. and Littlechild, R. (eds) (2000) *User Involvement and Participation in Social Care: Research informing practice*, Jessica Kingsley, London

Kemshall, H. and Littlechild, R. (2000) Research Informing Practice: Some concluding remarks. In Kemshall, H. and Littlechild, R. (eds) *User Involvement and Participation in Social Care: Research informing practice*, Jessica Kingsley, London

King, K. (1994) Method and Methodology in Feminist Research: What is the difference? *Journal of Advanced Nursing*, **20(1)**, 19–22

Kirk-Smith, M. (1996) Winning Ways With Research Proposals and Reports. *Nursing Times*, **92(11)**, 36–38

Kohler Riessman, C. (1993) *Narrative Analysis*, Sage, Thousand Oaks

Koluchova, J. (1976) Severe Deprivation in Twins: A case study. In Clarke, A. M. and Clarke, A. D. B. *Early Experience: myth and evidence*, Open Books, London

Kvale, S. (1996) *Interviews: An introduction to qualitative research interviewing*, Sage, London

Laidler, P. (1994) *Stroke Rehabilitation: Structure and strategy*, Chapman and Hall, London

Larson, E. A. and Fanchiang, S. C. (1996) Life History and Narrative Research: Generating a humanistic knowledge base for occupational therapy. *The American Journal of Occupational Therapy*, **50(4)**, 247–249

Lincoln, Y. S. and Guba, E. G. (2000) Paradigmatic Controversies, Contradictions, and Emerging Confluences. In Denzin, N. K. and Lincoln, Y. S. (eds) *Handbook of Qualitative Research* (2nd ed.), Sage, Thousand Oaks

Linstone, H. A. and Turoff, M. (eds) (1975) *The Delphi Method: Techniques and applications*, Addison-Wesley, Cambridge, Massachusetts

Lipson, J. G. (1997) The Politics of Publishing: Protecting participants' confidentiality. In Morse J. M. (ed) *Completing a Qualitative Project: Details and dialogue*, Sage, Thousand Oaks

Lister, R. (1999) Loss of Ability to Drive Following a Stroke: The early experiences of three elderly people on discharge from hospital. *British Journal of Occupational Therapy*, **62(11)**, 514–520

Lloyd, M., Preston-Shoot, M., Temple, B. and Wuu, R. (1996) Whose Project is it Anyway? Sharing and shaping the research and development agenda. *Disability and Society*, **11(3)**, 301–315

Mahat, G. (1997) Perceived Stressors and Coping Strategies Among Individuals with Rheumatoid Arthritis. *Journal of Advanced Nursing*, 25(6), 1144–1150

Maisel, R. and Persell, C. H. (1996) *How Sampling Works*, Pine Forge Press, Thousand Oaks

Mannerkorpi, K., Kroksmark, T. and Ekdahl, C. (1999) How Patients with Fibromyalgia Experience Their Symptoms in

Everyday Life. *Physiotherapy Research International*, **4(2)**, 110–122

Marshall, C. and Rossman G. (1995) *Designing Qualitative Research* (2nd ed.), Sage, London

Martlew, B. (1996) What Do You Let the Patient Tell You? *Physiotherapy*, **82(10)**, 558–565

Mason, J. (1996) *Qualitative Researching*, Sage, London

Mattingly, C. (1991) The Narrative Nature of Clinical Reasoning. *American Journal of Occupational Therapy*, **45**, 998–1005

Mattingly, C. and Gillette, N. (1991) Anthropology, Occupational Therapy and Action Research. *American Journal of Occupational Therapy*, **45(11)**, 972–978

May, T. (1997) *Social Research: Issues, method and process* (2nd ed.), Open University Press, Buckingham

McCall, J. (1996) *Statistics: A guide for therapists*, Butterworth-Heinemann, Oxford

McCarthy, I. C. (1994) Poverty: An invitation to colonial practice? *Feedback*, **3**, 17–21

Mcintyre, A. (1999) Elderly fallers: A baseline audit of admissions to a day hospital for elderly people. *British Journal of Occupational Therapy*, **62(6)**, 244–248

McKay, E. A. and Ryan, S. (1995) Clinical Reasoning Through Story Telling: Examining a student's case story on fieldwork placement. British Journal of Occupational Therapy, **58**, 234–238

Melton, J. (1998) How Do Clients with Learning Disabilities Evaluate Their Experience of Cooking with the Occupational Therapist? *British Journal of Occupational Therapy*, **61(3)**, 106–110

Miller, W. L. (1994) Common Space: Creating a collaborative research conversation. In Crabtree, B. F., Miller, W. L., Addison, R. B. *et al* (eds) *Exploring Collaborative Research in Primary Care*, Sage, London

Morra, M. E. (1984) How to Plan and Carry Out Your Poster Session, *Oncology Nursing Forum*, **11(2)**, 52–57

Morris, T. and Morris, C. (1995) The Image of Physiotherapy as Portrayed in Advertisements. *Physiotherapy*, **81(5)**, 293–294

Morse, J. (1994) 'Emerging from the Data': The cognitive processes of analysis in qualitative inquiry. In Morse, J. M. (ed)

Critical Issues in Qualitative Research Methods, Sage, Thousand Oaks

Munin, M., Rudy, T., Glynn, N., Crossett, L. and Rubash, H. (1998) Early Inpatient Rehabilitation After Elective Hip and Knee Arthroplasty. *The Journal of the American Medical Association*, **279(11)**, 847–852

Munson, R. (1996) *Intervention and Reflection: Basic issues in medical ethics* (5th ed.), Wadsworth Publication Co., Belmont, California

Murray, R. (1998) Measurement of the Effect of Participation in a Medical Humanities Group on the Practice of Physiotherapists. *Physiotherapy*, **84(10)**, 473–479

National Centre for Clinical Audit (1997) *NCCA Criteria for Clinical Audit*, BMA House, NCCA, London

Naylor, M. D. (1990) Special Feature: An Example of a Research Grant Application: Comprehensive discharge planning for the elderly. *Research in Nursing & Health*, **13(5)**, 327–347

Neville, S. and French, S. (1991) Clinical Education: Students' and clinical educators' views. *Physiotherapy*, **77(5)**, 351–354

Nochi, M (1998) Struggling with the Labelled Self: People with traumatic brain injuries in social settings. *Qualitative Health Research*, **8(5)**, 665–681

Oja, S. N. and Smulyan, L. (1989) *Collaborative Action Research: A developmental approach*, The Falmer Press, Lewes

Okihiro, G. Y. (1981) Oral History and the Writing of Ethnic History. In Perks, R. and Thomson, A. (eds) *The Oral History Reader*, Routledge, London

Olesen, V. (1998) Feminisms and Models of Qualitative Research. In Denzin, N. K. and Lincoln, Y. S. (eds) *The Landscape of Qualitative Research*, Sage, Thousand Oaks

Oliver, M. (1992) Changing the Social Relations of Research Production. *Disability, Handicap and Society*, **7(2)**, 101–114

Onions, C. T. (1966) *Oxford Dictionary of English Etymology*, Clarendon Press, Oxford

Parr, S. and Byng, S. with Ireland, C. (1996) *Talking About Aphasia: Living with loss of language after stroke*, Open University Press, Buckingham

Patton, M. Q. (1990) *Qualitative Evaluation and Research Methods* (2nd ed.), Sage, London

Phillips, E. M. and Pugh, D. S. (1994) *How To Get A PhD: A handbook for students and their supervisors*, Open University Press, Buckingham

Pietroni, P. C. (1994) Interprofessional Teamwork: Its history and development in hospitals, general practice and community care (UK). In Leathard, A. (ed) *Going Interprofessional: Working together for health and welfare*, Routledge, London

Polgar, S. and Thomas, S. A. (1995) *Introduction to Research in the Health Sciences* (3rd ed.), Churchill Livingstone, Edinburgh

Ponsford, A. and French, S. (1989) The Man Nobody Thought Could Drive. *Therapy Weekly*, **15(40)**, 9

Prentice, E. D. and Purtilo, R. B. (1993) The Use and Protection of Human and Animal Subjects. In Bork, C. E. (ed) *Research in Physical Therapy*, J. B. Lippincott Company, Philadelphia

Pritchard, P. and Pritchard, J. (1992) *Developing Team Work in Primary Healthcare: A practical workbook*, Oxford Medical Publications, Oxford

Punch, K. F. (1998) *Introduction to Social Research: Quantitative and qualitative approaches*, Sage, London

Punch, M. (1994) Politics and Ethics in Qualitative Research. In Denzin, N. K. and Lincoln, Y. S. (eds) *Handbook of Qualitative Research*, Sage, Thousand Oaks

Reason, P. (ed) (1994) *Participation in Human Inquiry*, Sage, London

Reason, P. and Heron, J. (1986) Research with People: The paradigm of co-operation experiential enquiry. *Person-Centred Review*, **1(4)**, 456–476

Redfern, S. J. and Norman, I. J. (1996) Clinical Audit, Related Cycles and Types of Health Care Quality: A preliminary model. *International Journal for Quality in Health Care*, **8(4)**, 331–340

Reed, J. and Biott, C. (1995) Evaluating and Developing Practitioner Research. In Reed, J. and Procter, S. (eds) *Practitioner Research in Health Care*, Chapman and Hall, London

Reynolds, F. A. (1996a) Evaluating the Impact of an Interprofessional Communication Course through Essay Content Analysis: Do physiotherapy and occupational therapy students' essays place similar emphasis on responding skills? *Journal of Interprofessional Care*, **10(3)**, 285–295

Reynolds, F. (1996b) Working with Movement as a Metaphor:

Understanding the therapeutic impact of physical exercise from a Gestalt perspective. *Counselling Psychology Quarterly*, **9(4)**, 383–390

Rosenhan, D. L. (1973) On Being Sane in Insane Places. *Science*, **179**, 250–258

Rubin, H. J. and Rubin, I. S. (1995) *Qualitative Interviewing: The art of hearing data*, Sage, Thousand Oaks

Sapsford, R. and Abbott, P. (1996) Ethics, Politics and Research. In Sapsford, R. and Jupp, V. (eds) *Data Collection and Analysis*, Sage, London

Schofield, W. (1996) Survey Sampling. In Sapsford, R. and Jupp, V. (eds) *Data Collection and Analysis*, Sage Publications, London

Schön, D. (1983) *The Reflective Practitioner*, Basic Books, New York

Schon, D. (1993) Reflection in Action. In Walmsley, J., Reynolds, J., Shakespeare, P. and Woolfe, R. (eds) *Health, Welfare and Practice: Reflecting on roles and relationships*, Sage, London

Scott, J. (1990) *A Matter of Record*, Polity Press, Cambridge

Seale, C. (1999) *The Quality of Qualitative Research*, London, Sage

Seale, J. and Barnard, S. (1998) *Therapy Research: Processes and practicalities*, Butterworth-Heinemann, Oxford

Sealey, C. (1999) Two Common Pitfalls in Clinical Audit: Failing to complete the audit cycle and confusing audit with research. *British Journal of Occupational Therapy*, **62(6)**, 238–243

Seymour, W. (1998) *Remaking the Body: Rehabilitation and change*, London, Routledge

Sieber, J. E. (1993) The Ethics and Politics of Sensitive Research. In Renzettl, C. and Lee, R. M. (eds) *Researching Sensitive Topics*, Sage, London

Silverman, D. (2000) *Doing Qualitative Research: A practical handbook*, Sage, London

Sim, J. (1989) Methodology and Morality in Physiotherapy Research. *Physiotherapy*, **75(4)**, 237–243

Sim, J. (1997) *Ethical Decision Making in Therapy Practice*, Butterworth-Heinemann, Oxford

Sim, J. and Snell, J. (1996) Focus Groups in Physiotherapy Evaluation and Research. *Physiotherapy*, **82(3)**, 189–198

Skeat, W. (1978) *An Etymological Dictionary of the English Language* (4th ed.), Oxford, Clarendon Press

Smith, S. (1996) Ethnographic Enquiry in Physiotherapy Research. 1. Illuminating the working culture of the physiotherapy assistant. *Physiotherapy*, **82(6)**, 342–348

Smith, J. and Topping, M. (1996) The Introduction of a Robotic Aid to Drawing into a School for Physically Handicapped Children: A case study. *Journal of Occupational Therapy*, **59(12)**, 565–569,

Smith, S. K. (2000) Sensitive Issues in Life Story Research. In Moch, S. D. and Gates, M. F. (eds) *The Researcher Experience in Qualitative Research*, Sage, Thousand Oaks

Somers, M. (1994) The Narrative Construction of Identity: A relational and network approach. *Theory and Society*, **23**, 606–649

Stake, R. E. (1995) *The Art of Case Study Research*, Sage, London

Stalker, K. (1998) Some Ethical and Methodological Issues in Research with People with Learning Difficulties. *Disability and Society*, **13(1)**, 5–19

Stanfield, J. H. (1998) Ethnic Modeling in Qualitative Research. In Denzin, N. K. and Lincoln, Y. S. (eds) *The Landscape of Qualitative Research*, Sage, Thousand Oaks

Stewart, D. W. and Shamdasani, P. N. (1990) *Focus Groups*, Sage, London

Strand, L. and Wie, S. (1999) The Sock Test for Evaluating Activity Limitation in Patients with Musculoskeletal Pain. *Physical Therapy*, **79(2)**, 136–145

Strauss, A. and Corbin, J. (1990) *Basics of Qualitative Research: Grounded theory procedures and techniques*, Sage, London

Sturgens, J. (1999) A Structure for Recording Qualitative Observation Associated with a Paediatric Assessment. *British Journal of Occupational Therapy*, **62(12)**, 543–548

Sumsion, T. (1999) A Study to Determine a British Occupational Therapy Definition of Client-Centred Practice. *British Journal of Occupational Therapy*, **62(2)**, 52–58

Swain, J. (1995) *The Use of Counselling Skills: A guide for therapists*, Butterworth-Heinemann, Oxford

Swain, J., Gillman, M. and French, S. (1998) *Confronting Disabling Barriers: Towards making organisations accessible*, Venture Press, Birmingham

Swenson, M. (1996) Research Briefs: Essential elements in a qualitative dissertation proposal. *Journal of Nursing Education*, **35(4)**, 188–190

Taylor, A. (1999) Physiological Response to a Short Period of Exercise Training in Patients with Chronic Heart Failure. *Physiotherapy Research International*, **4(4)**, 237–249

Teram, E., Schachter, C. L. and Stalker, C. A. (1999) Opening the Doors to Disclosure: Childhood sexual abuse survivors reflect on telling physiotherapists about their trauma. *Physiotherapy*, **85(2)**, 88–97

Tesch, R. (1990) *Qualitative Research: Analysis types and software tools*, Falmer, London

Thomas, C. and Parry, A. (1996) Research on Users' Views about Stroke Services: Towards an empowerment research paradigm or more of the same? *Physiotherapy*, **82(1)**, 6–12

Thomas, K., Fitter, M., Brazier, J. *et al* (1999) Longer-Term Clinical and Economic Benefits of Offering Acupuncture to Patients with Chronic Low Back Pain Assessed as Suitable for Primary Care Management. *Complementary Therapies in Medicine*, **7(2)**, 91–100

Thompson, N. (1996) *People Skills: A Guide to effective practice in the human services*, Macmillan Press, Houndmills

Thompson, N. (1998) *Promoting Equality: Challenging discrimination and oppression in the human services*, Macmillan, Houndmills

Thompson, P. (2000) The Development of Oral History in Britain. In Bornat, J., Parks, R., Thompson, P. and Walmsley, J. (eds) *Oral History, Health and Welfare*, Routledge, London

Thower, N. (1990) *Standing on the Shoulders of Giants: A longer view of Newton and Halley*, University of California Press

Trainor, A. and Ezer, H. (2000) Rebuilding Life: The experience of living with AIDS after facing imminent death. *Qualitative Health Research*, **10(5)**, 646–660

Tripp-Reimer, T., Sorofman, B., Peters, J. and Waterman, J. E. (1994) Research Teams: Possibilities and pitfalls in collaborative qualitative research. In Morse, J. M. (ed) *Critical Issues in Qualitative Research Methods*, Sage, Thousand Oaks

Tryssenaar, J. (1999) The Lived Experience of Becoming an Occupational Therapist. *British Journal of Occupational Therapy*, **82(3)**, 107–111

Tyson, S. F. and Turner, G. F. (1999) Southampton Stroke Audit:

Assessing service quality. *British Journal of Therapy & Rehabilitation*, **6(5)**, 227–232

Uzzell, D. (1995) Ethnographic and Action Research. In Breakwell, G., Hammond, S. and Fife-Schaw, C. (eds) *Research Methods in Psychology*, Sage, London

Walmsley, J. (1998) Life History Interviews with People with Learning Disabilities. In Perks, R. and Thomson, A. (eds) *The Oral History Reader*, Routledge, London

Walmsley, J. and Atkinson, D. (2000) Oral History and the History of Learning Disability. In Bornat, J., Parks, R., Thompson, P. and Walmsley, J. (eds) *Oral History, Health and Welfare*, Routledge, London

Weerakoon, P. and O'Sullivan, V. (1998) Inappropriate Patient Sexual Behaviour in Physiotherapy Practice. *Physiotherapy*, **84(10)**, 401–499

Weindling, A., Hallam, P., Gregg, J. *et al* (1996) A Randomised Controlled Trial of Early Physiotherapy for High-Risk Infants. *Acta Paediatrica*, **85(9)**, 1107–1111

Widdershoven, G. A. M. and Smits, M. -J. (1996) Ethics and Narratives. In Josselson, R. (ed) *Ethics and Process in the Narrative Study of Lives*, Sage, Thousand Oaks

Widdershoven, G. A. M. (1993) The Story of Life; Hermeneutic perspectives on the relationship between narrative and life history. In Josselson, R. and Lieblich, A. (eds) *The Narrative Story of Lives*, Sage, Thousand Oaks

Williams, A. (1997) Pitfalls on the Road to Ethical Approval. *Nurse Researcher*, **5(1)**, 15–22

Wilson, H. S. and Hutchinson, S. A. (1997) Presenting Qualitative Research Up Close: Visual literacy in poster presentations. In Morse, J. M. (ed) *Completing a Qualitative Project: Details and dialogue*, Sage, Thousand Oaks

Yin, R. K. (1994) *Case Study Research* (2nd ed.), Sage, London

Zarb, G. (1992) On the Road to Damascus: First steps towards changing the relations of research production, *Disability, Handicap and Society*, **7(2)**, 125–138

Index